Forward

Thank you for purchasing "Eat Stop And Eat"! We hope you glean some valuable information within these pages. Information that could make you feel better, and live a longer and healthier life!

This book is dedicated to a generation of people who have tried and failed, many times over, to keep their weight under control by following fad diets and other false direction from so-called experts.

Eat Stop And Eat

By Faron Connelly

Introduction

The secret to losing weight, and keeping it off, is quite simple; the less we consume, the less we will weigh. And, if we keep our food intake monitored and at a level that is most productive to our systems, the better we will feel, and the healthier we will be. But, we all know that easing back your food intake can be a real challenge–easier said than done.

About a decade ago, I began observing our aging population and noticed one thing that the healthier group of seniors had in common; they were noticeably slim. It is a rarity to see an 80 year-old man or woman who is obese. Our bodies are not designed to function efficiently with excess weight to pack around. I once read an article published by the L.A. Times back in 2014, which reveals some startling facts about obesity:

"Those with a body mass index, or BMI, above 40 are robbed of at least 6 1/2 years, on average, of expected life span, a study has found. And the toll in years lost rises "with the degree of obesity, reaching nearly 14 years for the most obese -- those with a BMI above 55, researchers said.

The study found that the reduction in life expectancy,

associated with being extremely obese, was similar to that seen in adults who smoke. And as a person's obesity rises to higher levels, his or her expected life span falls below that of smokers. The findings come from a project that aggregated the results of about 20 long-term studies on obesity conducted in the United States, Australia and Sweden. They were published in the journal PLoS Medicine, in what is believed to be the largest study to date of the health consequences of severe obesity.

Compared with their normal-weight peers, the extremely obese are more likely to succumb early to heart disease, cancer and diabetes. For men with "class III obesity," the rate of death attributable to heart disease and diabetes is especially elevated compared with normal-weight males. For women in the same obesity category, cancer deaths dramatically outstripped those among normal-weight women. But premature deaths attributable to all causes, from injury to chronic lower respiratory infections, were consistently higher in those with severe obesity, the study found. The extremely obese -- those who generally would need to lose 100 pounds. or more to attain a "normal healthy weight" -- are a fast-growing segment of the U.S. population, now representing about 6% of American adults". The ranks of those with a BMI over 40 (for example, a 5-foot-6 person weighing 250 pounds or more) have grown fourfold since the 1980s. The population with a BMI over 50 (say, a 5-foot-10 person weighing more than 350 pounds) has grown by 10% in the same period. Simply put, obesity will shorten your life. I'm glad you've decided to pick up this book, and I hope that you will glean something from it, which will motivate you to succeed in keeping fit and living a long and healthy life. You deserve it, and your family deserves it.

Cheers,

Faron Connelly

About Fasting and Weight Loss

An intermittent fasting diet is one of the best ways to help you lose weight fast! Alternatively, fasting incorrectly can be a very unhealthy choice. For the past decade or so, many fad diets have been pushed down our throats. They tell us that there is now a new "miracle method" of losing weight fast. WRONG! If you want to improve your body, your self-esteem, and become all-around healthier, intermittent fasting is a great way to go! It is safe and effective. In this book, you are going to discover why this type of fasting is the perfect means to help you get stronger too!

You will learn how making this a "lifestyle change", can improve your health dramatically... and in so many ways! You'll have more energy and endurance than you've had in a long, long time. So put away the diet pills, and get ready to learn something that can literally save your life.

What Exactly Is Intermittent Fasting Anyway?

Intermittent fasting is simply time-restricted eating to help an individual remain healthy by reducing excess fat in their body. It involves a person cycling between a state of fasting (fasted) and non-fasting (fed) state. The person chooses to take periodic breaks from eating, during which they may take part in resistance exercises such as weight lifting or cardio exercises. The periodic breaks from eating can be very flexible and may range from 12 to 24 hours, once, twice or more times every week.

Right from the onset, it is critical to note that this is not a diet program. Intermittent fasting does not involve phasing, point systems, or weighing of food and there are no foods that are off-limits.

In the intermittent fasting nutritional custom lifestyle, fasts can be combined with resistance training routines such as lifting weights and cardio exercises. This combination makes losing excess fat easier and more sustainable in the long term. For the "Eat Stop Eat" lifestyle (a form of intermittent fasting), a 24-hour fasting period is recommended, although 16 to 20 hour periods also work. Intermittent fasting (IF) and caloric restriction (CR), are two forms of dietary restriction (DR). Intermittent fasting requires changing your dietary patterns, and simply choosing to eat meals during different times of the day. You're still going to get to eat the things you like, but you'll learn to eat them differently than you used to.

This diet (more accurately - fast) will naturally help you lose weight, making you feel better, stronger, and much healthier for life! People, who succeed with (IF), find themselves re-energized. One simple reason for this is because of how well fasting removes fat and toxins. Caloric restriction is something that a wise person will practice daily - even if weight is not an issue. Some refer to it as dietary restriction, or portion control. Intermittent fasting is simply another way of interpreting CR. Fasting essentially is "The willful act of abstaining from food (and in some cases drink), for a pre-determined period of time". That's right, a predetermined period of time. I hope to convince you that making the mindful decision, and setting a goal for yourself, is the best way to succeed. This new habit can, and will, become a very natural way of life. Once you've set your routine - allowing yourself meal times when you've made the predetermined schedule, it will feel quite natural!

Once new habits are formed, intermittent fasting, improved health, and weight loss become synonymous!

Is Intermittent Fasting Safe?

Short Answer: Yes. Fasting is the simplest method our body has for maintaining its caloric balance. It's okay to take the occasional break from eating – now and again Some might say that it is very difficult to practice this kind of regimen, or that depriving your body of food is unhealthy. However, recent studies suggest otherwise!

Naturally, if you're experiencing any pre-existing health issues, you should consult with your physician. IF (intermittent fasting - is what we'll be referring to) is a method which should be practiced "by the book". Don't go it alone. There are many resources available to you. Feedback received from the millions who practice intermittent fasting, say that this type of fasting is really easy to do – once you get used to it. It typically takes less than a week to become comfortable with your new eating schedule. It is completely safe, and people would not likely continue if it wasn't a really good option for their bodies; making them feel stronger, healthier, and all around, better... and bi-annual checkups with their doctor have confirmed results."

People struggle with trying to maintain health, strength, and longevity... we all fight weight gain as we age, and get less exercise. But it doesn't have to be this way! If you really want to get healthy, then this diet is safe to try, and it may be for you. Along with exercise, it is a great way to become healthier and stronger, in a relatively short amount of time. Oh, and by the way... and save money at the grocer.

* * *

All this said, intermittent fasting is not the only option available. Other "diets" are available, but you must be willing and able to develop, and stick to, an exercise routine – an intense physical workout is great! But, unfortunately we know there are some of us with physical ailments (arthritis, for example) that are not able to perform some of the most basic exercise routines. ...Intermittent fasting to the rescue! After shedding a few pounds, you might find yourself easing into an exercise program. Physical movement becomes less stressful on the body.

Fasting takes time to get comfortable with. If this sounds impossible to accomplish, please consider the alternatives – staying "just the way you are". Great health, and a great life are worth making some sacrifices. Start out by taking it slowly, and working your way up. The stomach may very well shrink somewhat, and the hunger cravings may subside. It's a mental game, as well! When you start seeing the pounds fall off, you'll be that much more determined to continue with the plan! You may become one of the millions that strongly attest to the results of intermittent fasting.

The Philosophy Behind IF

The obesity and weight problems that are happening in the United States are not caused by the intake of only sugar or fat. In truth, obesity is not developed through having an abundance of just one specific macronutrient in our diets. The number one cause of obesity is the abundance of food. Basically, there is just too much food available for consumption.

Statistics indicate that every single day, the food industry in the United States produces food that is enough to supply every person in the United States with approximately 4000 calories. 4000 calories is almost twice of what a single person typically needs in a day.

Part of the obesity problem is that we keep looking in the wrong places for answers. Diet is a very small part of the cause of obesity when compared to the abundance of food in the market. The combination of an efficient, relentless food marketing industry and a misleading health and nutrition industry have led to the current obesity epidemic in the United States. Simply put, most people in the US eat too much and yet most of them have no idea why.

Intermittent fasting (short breaks from eating) is the perfect solution to the abundance problem. The food industry will undoubtedly continue producing more and more food, therefore helping the consumers to develop the self- discipline of "Eat Stop Eat" will create a sustainable model of regulating fat intake.

With intermittent fasting you do not have to impose restrictions on yourself for foods that you like, all you have to do is commit to keep from eating solid food for short periods once or several times per week. For those who might be thinking that this is impossible, consider this – you already fast for around 6 to 10 hours every night when sleeping. Intermittent fasting involves expanding that time frame for a bit longer for sustainable weight loss.

You do not need to worry if you are unable to fast for 24 hours every time. 24 hours was simply chosen since it is an easy enough time-frame to remember. It also allows people to eat every day, and is appropriate for various levels of weight loss needs. If 24 hours is too hard for you, then you can try 16 or 20 hours. The most important thing is that you are taking significant short breaks from eating. During these fasting periods, you can commit to resistance training in order to achieve better results.

* * *

I recall a high-school friend of mine by the name of Brad. Brad was a big boy, a football star, and feared by many. Yes, he was a great high-school linebacker (and boy, could he mow the other players off the field). He fed his big frame and football game, almost continuously. At that age, our appetites and hormones race wildly. We require nutrients to keep us going, and to sustain our level of energy – but, not Jolly Ranchers and Chips!

As Brad's body matured in height, his weight became a serious issue. You see, his metabolism began to slow rapidly after his teen years, but his appetite did not. In his 20's, Brad still ate like a teenaged linebacker. He was the product of an environment in which so many of us were raised. Brad had developed eating habits early on, which at the time, suited his passion for football. His mother made sure he was "well-fed", by preparing meals, always served on time. She usually prepared twice as much food for the family as was necessary, or needed. The fridge was always stocked and openly available for Brad. For kids growing up in the 70's, this was the norm.

Once Brad graduated and took a job at the local newspaper office, he began to really put on the pounds. He would snack between meals, and be the first one out the door for his lunch break. By 30 years of age, Brad was obese. He began suffering issues with breathing, which eventually led to regular doctor visits and consultations about weight, heart issues, and the likeliness of diabetes to follow. Not long after Brad was given a dim prognosis from his doctor, I met up with him. I told Brad that I had always been a fan, and was sorry to hear about his issue with weight gain and health. Brad asked me what I was doing to keep in shape and why some people gain weight more quickly than others. "It isn't fair", he murmured. This was an open door and opportunity for me to tell Brad about what I've discovered about intermittent fasting!

I presented Brad with an idea. "What if you could still eat the things you like, and lose weight at the same time" I said. He looked at me as though I didn't really have a clue about his condition. "Hear me out" I replied. I then proceeded to tell him how losing weight could be accomplished by implementing the oldest, and simplest technique known to man - Stop eating momentarily - take a break - then another - then start eating again! I painted a picture for him of the olden days when farmers would be out working in the fields all day long without eating, and how primitive man only ate when he was able to find wild game for sustenance.

"Brad was intrigued with the idea, but wasn't sure how it would work for him. "I'm always hungry, and chronically fatigued" he said. I went on to explain the benefits of intermittent fasting, and how I was sure that it could help with his weight and lack of energy. Brad was fearful of his poor health, and told me that he would be willing to give anything a try. "I have two little girls that need me" he said. Later that evening, I emailed Brad a digital copy of a book that I had read about Caloric Restriction, and the many benefits of intermittent fasting. My hope and intent was to encourage him - by educating him.

I was delighted to hear back from Brad 12 months later. He was ecstatic and wanted to share with me that he had implemented a fasting regimen, his health had dramatically improved, and that he had lost almost 55 pounds! This was one of the most rewarding moments of my life.

The Science Behind Intermittent Fasting

Basically, our human bodies are designed to effortlessly transition between the "Fed" and "Fasted" state. During the fed state, the levels of insulin in the body are elevated, which has the effect of signaling our bodies to store excess calories in our fat cells. With insulin present, the body stops burning fat and instead burns glucose from the last meal that we ate.

During the fasted state, insulin levels drop while glucagon and other growth hormones which oppose insulin are elevated. In this state, the body begins to mobilize and burn the fat (instead of glucose) that had been stored in our fat cells, so as to produce energy.

The bottom-line is that with intermittent fasting, you can burn off fat by simply not eating for short periods of time. You can then resume eating after each fast in order to achieve a healthy metabolic balance between the fed and fasted state.

Benefits of Intermittent Fasting

Intermittent fasting is the best and simplest way to lose weight, maintain muscles and experience all the wonderful health benefits that come as a result of fasting. It does not require any complex nutritional planning. This method does not require any special shopping trips, exotic foods or costly supplements. It simply requires that you desist from eating for short period(s) each week.

It is also the most stress-free way of getting rid of obsessive compulsive eating habits and the constant need to browse through magazine pages and the Internet in a bid to get the latest and best diet program or strategy.

With intermittent fasting, you will be able to break away from the compulsion and guilt that propels so many of today's eating habits. Intermittent fasting does away with the idea that you have to be constantly eating or that there is only one true and perfect way of eating.

One of the great advantages that intermittent fasting has over diet plans is that it is highly adaptable and flexible which makes it more sustainable compared to diet plans. This flexibility makes it a sustainable addition to the way people eat for the rest of their lives. This allows people to follow it as they successfully lose weight and keep the weight off, long after losing it.

It is simply the easiest and most flexible way to lose fat, keep fit and maintain a trim body. In fact all you are doing is allowing your body to lose fat by doing nothing. You are not cooking, eating and most importantly you are not worrying about what you are eating. In addition, you don't have to go a day without eating!

* * *

It works very much like this; you start your day with a simple breakfast, then lunch at noon. Later, have a very light dinner in the early evening, and drink plenty of water - a lot of water. With time, dinner goes away... completely. There is no longer a need for a large dinner – and seeing yourself losing weight, will only drive you forward. If you can make it through the last several hours of the day without eating, you'll afterwards, be adding an additional eight hours of fasting while you sleep. Once you've made the choice to skip a single dinner, you will have fasted from noon to breakfast the following day – that could be upwards of a 20 hour fast! The fact is, many people lose a ton of weight just by avoiding dinner alone. As long as you stick with a diet that follows this general method of fasting, you WILL lose a lot of natural weight, guaranteed. It only stands to reason–if you eat less during the day, you will weigh less in the long run... not rocket science. But there is more involved in eating correctly (we'll get to that later). A lot of cultures consume far less (daily), than those of us in other parts of the world. We have been "programmed" to prepare and to eat three meals per day. Eating has become a "social event". Some folks wake up in the morning, planning what they will be having for dinner! Breakfast, lunch, and dinner have long been the standard diet – especially for those of us living in the U.S.

As you may know, modern day knowledge of intermittent fasting has come a long way. Now, widespread recognition of this practice is showing many individuals, scientists and physicians the benefits. Mainstream fitness authorities concur with the IF benefits gained for health, fitness and wellbeing. Studies, like one performed by Dr. Mark, clearly prove that other mammals (such as mice) obtained an increased lifespan, along with improvement in major health indicators; these include body composition, insulin sensitivity, and Nero-regeneration capacity. There are many variables when it comes to intermittent fasting. As with any nutritional, exercise program, or new routine, a "one size fits all" advice is not usually considered prudent.

Many variations for intermittent fasting can be recommended; fasting every other day, all day, twice per week, every third day, once every other week, and so-on.

Some lighter diets advise skipping dinner, or skipping breakfast. You'll also hear recommendations such us "eat only when you feel hungry" or "don't eat if you don't feel hungry". This practice has been particularly well received among various religious faiths, with sound results.

Education Is Key

The scientific community utilizes many resources to find the quantitative proof for intermittent fasting benefits, and the results speak for themselves. Many health benefits can be derived. Obese individuals, searching for treatment, which does not involve dangerous drugs, chemicals, and sometimes life-threatening surgery, have achieved the most prolific results. The advice of skipping a meal or a series of meals goes against popular culture beliefs, since our culture suggests eating three substantial meals per day. Some obese people owe their health problems to these generalized cultural beliefs!

Many people associate the act of fasting with unpleasantness, and no likely visible benefits; but as scientific research progresses, people are learning that the benefits of intermittent fasting are increasing lifespan considerably, reducing unhealthy weight, and improving self-determination and worth. Evidence shows that many yogis in India, and practitioners from around the world, live a surprisingly long life, due to the single fact that they eat much less than people in other parts of the world. This phenomenon has been investigated thoroughly and it seems that there will be much more to come about intermittent fasting and the outstanding benefits.

Obviously, considerations should be taken when it comes to fasting; i.e., pregnant women, and individuals with glucose level related diseases, should abstain from the practice for health reasons. Caloric restriction (CR) itself, is the best way to keep body weight within an acceptable "fat to muscle ratio", and it is one of the most important factors to help reduce heart and age related illness. Other benefits such as avoiding cognitive decline (dementia), improving resistance to cancer, and improving quality of life, should be enough to motivate any individual to at least try intermittent fasting. Medical research for this subject is in its infancy, and is already showing promising results .

More Benefits Of "IF"

Intermittent fasting is the best and simplest way to lose weight, maintain muscles and experience all the wonderful health benefits that come as a result of fasting. It does not require any complex nutritional planning. This method does not require any special shopping trips, exotic foods or costly supplements. It simply requires that you desist from eating for short period(s) each week.

It is also the most stress-free way of getting rid of obsessive compulsive eating habits and the constant need to browse through magazine pages and the Internet in a bid to get the latest and best diet program or strategy.

With intermittent fasting, you will be able to break away from the compulsion and guilt that propels so many of today's eating habits. Intermittent fasting does away with the idea that you have to be constantly eating or that there is only one true and perfect way of eating.

One of the great advantages that intermittent fasting has over diet plans is that it is highly adaptable and flexible which makes it more sustainable compared to diet plans. This flexibility makes it a sustainable addition to the way people eat for the rest of their lives. This allows people to follow it as they successfully lose weight and keep the weight off, long after losing it. It is simply the easiest and most flexible way to lose fat, keep fit and maintain a trim body. In fact all you are doing is allowing your body to lose fat by doing nothing. You are not cooking, eating and most importantly you are not worrying about what you are eating. In addition, you don't have to go a day without eating.

* * *

Many who take up weight loss programs, at one time or another, hear about intermittent fasting. The discovery often comes about when they are looking for alternative ways of dealing with excessive body weight and health issues. If you are researching the benefits of IF, and want to learn basic applications, then read on. You will find out why intermittent fasting is good for your health and body, and for weight training. The medically sound fast should be conducted for 24-36 hours. You can do this once a week, if you have a difficult time fasting at work. For those who have relatively few work commitments, and an open schedule, three times per week would be great! The increased number of fasts allows you to reduce the duration of each individual fast, and you still reap the benefits. Here is a simple methodology of intermittent fasting that you can apply immediately: *Eat breakfast on day one. The next meal you eat should be on the following day*. If you find out that this practice is not physically possible in your case, vary the mealtime or the duration. But, push yourself as far as you can. It takes trial and error, to find out what works best for you. Do what you'll be able to do and to stick to doing! Don't let despair or habitual "three-squares- a-day" eating keep you from testing possible combinations of meal times and/or the duration of your fast. Although this can be relatively easy, it will require some effort on your part. The changes you see and feel after just a couple of weeks, far outweigh the effort.

When you first begin intermittent fasting, you force your body to use its internal food reserves for energy and other metabolic processes. As it consumes food reserves, your body will also increase the rate at which it releases waste substances through your various body organs such as the skin, digestive system and lymph system. This is a process known as dysphagia. It encompasses the removal of various waste-matter from body cells throughout the body. One well-known benefit of taking up this method of fasting is that it assists your body in defending itself from Alzheimer's disease. You start to rid your body of toxins, and an increased production of the "brain-derived neurotropic factor (BDNF)" commences.

For people who are also into Paleo diets, the practice

of intermittent fasting leads to stimulation of growth. As long as you eat your normal amount of food before and after every fast, the period of BDNF will induce an increase in the production of growth hormones! Crazy, huh?

Weight Lifting: For many people who are weightlifting, this added benefit gives them faster results in increased muscle mass. It is important for everyone who is fasting to continue doing their daily activities, as if they were not fasting! Don't forget this crucial part of your progress.

This practice helps the body to maintain a metabolic balance, so instead of breaking down your muscles, it breaks down excess body fat. Before going ahead with your fast, you might consider talking to your nutritionist to get advice about the adequate amount of calories and other food quantities you need for optimum functionality of YOUR body, as each of us have different metabolisms.

* * *

Vital benefits = Prolonging of life. When it comes to intermittent fasting, there are a number of crucial aspects that must be taken into consideration. Intermittent fasting is not a starvation process, or some sort of fad diet. It is a healthy eating plan. When someone fasts, they simply lower their daily calorie intake. This is proven to help lead a healthier, happier, and extended life! As an example, you may know that our ancestors were basically hunters and gatherers. They didn't always have food readily available, and mealtime was totally dependent on what nature provided – at that particular time, or season. Now, this means that the human body is designed to remain fully functional for some time – without food intake! The body has plenty of fuel to last without consuming three meals per day. What follows, are a few examples of intermittent fasting health benefits.

By following an intermittent eating schedule, you will have more energy – As you will not be eating much, the wavering of blood sugar levels will be lessened. This process will ensure that real energy is consistent. You'll be lighter on your feet. Also, it will help you lower the risk of developing diabetes. You still need to make sure to exercise on regular basis while you are fasting, as it will enhance your body's abilities to consume more fats. Your body releases a growth hormone during fasting, which helps your body to consume more calories.

As you burn more fats, the pounds begin to drop. And, due to the fact that you are eating less calories, your body will start consuming excessive body fat... instead of getting energy from food that you eat while following a "normal" eating plan. Your body thereby develops more lean muscle mass. If fasting is engaged for more than 12 hours, your body has already began consuming the body fat! ...12 hours. There are other incentives to get you excited about IF. Benefits include: less glucose in the blood, improved insulin levels, less inflammation (from gout or arthritis), and common safeguards against deadly diseases like cancer, heart disease, and Alzheimer's.

You can start a simple fast by opting for a one-day skip of breakfast. You may drink tea or water instead of having breakfast. When moving forward, try skipping lunch. If you need to eat more, then go ahead and have a full size meal. Remember, this is not like starvation, so it must be followed wisely. Keep your determination and willpower in check.

There is a common misconception that this way of eating is somewhat similar to starvation, which it is not! In fact, once adapted, intermittent fasting keeps you full. In this plan (when carrying out "IF"), ghrelin, a hormone which is responsible for hunger signals, makes adjustments to the new style of eating, thereby relieving you from hunger! Another efficient benefit of intermittent fasting, is that it increases concentration. During a fast, another hormone is produced, known as catecholamines. As a result, you become more focused. Very cool – wouldn't you say? But note: If you are seriously considering intermittent fasting, you should probably first seek the advice of your healthcare professional. The schedule above is merely a sample, or an example, of what you may consider setting up to start your regimen.

Common Forms Of Intermittent Fasting

Let's get into the practical and technical details of intermittent fasting. There are several common ways to practice intermittent fasting. We will look at three of the most common variations. All three of these involve extending the natural overnight fast period by not taking breakfast and pushing forward the first meal of the day.

All of these also comprise of taking no calories at the start of the day and then eating the majority of your calories later in the day, a concept that is referred to as a caloric "reverse taper".

For the purpose of discussing these forms of intermittent fasting, the baseline standard plan shall consists of 12 hours of fasting (overnight) and 12 hours of an eating window during the day which consists of 3 meals, that is, breakfast, lunch, and dinner.

Lean-gains

Lean-gains is an intermittent fasting method that was popularized by a bodybuilder by the name of Martin Berkhan, it is arguably the most popular method to date. This method of fasting involves skipping breakfast every fasting day and taking lunch as the first meal of the day. Essentially, you don't take breakfast and then you eat an ordinary lunch and dinner within an 8-hour window.

With this method, the general idea is to fast for at least 16 hours (the overnight 12 hours plus the first approximately 6 hours of the day) then take all the calories you need within an 8-hour feeding window.

For instance, you get up at 6:00 a.m. skip breakfast and eat nothing for 6 hours, and then you have your lunch at around noon and your dinner at 8:00 p.m. in the evening. In this method, taking snacks within the feeding window is allowed (although not advisable). Basically it is a 16:8 division of your 24 hours where you fast for 16 hours and eat within an 8-hour window every day. This method results in 4 hours of fasting every day above the 12-hour baseline natural overnight fasting.

Warrior Diet

The Warrior Diet was popularized by Ori Hofmekler. It involves fasting for the majority of your day, then taking all of the calories your body needs in the evening. The objective of this method is to go without breakfast and lunch, then feast on a huge dinner within a 4-hour window in the evening. This actually results in a 20:4 hour division where 20 hours are dedicated to fasting and the remaining 4 hours functions as a feeding window. This form of intermittent fasting allows you to enjoy very large and satisfying meals in the evening. It is perfect for someone who is going out for a social dinner where there is bound to be plenty of calorie- rich foods.

Fasting for such a long period during the day is actually more difficult but it leads to an in-depth level of fat adaptation and low insulin (which improves insulin sensitivity). Because of its intensity, you may choose to do it approximately 3 times a week. If you were to follow this plan, it would give you eight hours of fasting above the baseline, every day that you fast.

What To Do While Fasting

As stated earlier Eat Stop Eat is not a diet plan so it would be counterintuitive to give you a bunch of recipes, protein and calorie charts, and food combination instructions that most people refer to as the "best". This is basically what most diet books and magazines comprise of. The truth is that such recipes and instructions will be setting you up for the disinhibition effect talked about earlier and would lead you to inevitable failure in the end. Below are a few tips and tricks to help make your fasting periods a bit easier. During your fasts, thirst can often be mistaken for hunger; therefore, it is important to drink plenty of non-caloric liquids as you fast. Start your day in the morning by taking a large glass of water. You can then take black coffee or tea as your breakfast. During the day you may also partake of diet colas, avoid artificial sweeteners. However, a small amount of the sweeteners cannot sabotage your fast, in case you absolutely cannot do without them.

There have been a lot of false rumors that aspartame, an artificial sweetener, causes a huge increase in insulin production in the body. These rumors are not based on science and multiple scientific studies have shown that aspartame has no negative or adverse effect on growth hormones or insulin in the human body. All in all, it does no harm to just use natural sweeteners instead of artificial ones when you fast. This will keep your mind from worrying if this sweetener or that sweetener will sabotage your fast.

There has also been some buzz that tea, coffee and cola which contain caffeine cause large spikes in the body's insulin levels. While there are studies that indicate that a combination of caffeine and carbohydrates leads to increase in insulin production, there are no studies that indicate that caffeine alone without carbs can cause an increase in insulin levels.

Drinks such as tea and coffee cannot mess up your metabolism during your fasts. However, make sure you keep your level of intake of this drinks at the same level as you would if you weren't fasting. Remember, Eat Stop Eat is just a temporary method of breaking from your normal feeding habits not a reason to radically change how you eat or drink.

Another important thing to remember is that you should strive to remain busy even as you fast. The truth of the matter is that most people use food as some form of "bio- feedback". Food has become a mental stimulus for many, such that when they are bored, all they can think about to improve their mood is eating some snacks or food.

Let me ask you this, have you ever noticed how much you eat during a day that you considered to be extremely boring? I bet it is more than you normally eat. This is because we tend to replace mental stimulation with food stimulation. This is especially the case for those who work in offices and live a relatively sedentary lifestyle. That is why it is important to stay busy and try to make your day-to-day activities more diverse, exciting and engaging. Have you ever noticed how "time flies" when you are doing something that really excites you, you even forget that you had to eat at some point. This is essentially the thinking behind staying busy.

Of course not every minute or hour in your daily life can be exciting, some tasks may get monotonous in the office or you may have to wait for an appointment for a few hours. However the key here is "diversity", just like in the food you eat. Introduce variety in you day to day tasks to avoid getting bored which results in snacking.

Just because you are fasting does not mean that you get to change your daily schedule or habits. Simply go about your daily activities just like any other normal day, let your metabolism deal with the internal changes and keep your mind from over-thinking your fasts. This is actually the beauty of Eat Stop Eat, you can go about your daily routine; shop, work, exercise, all the while losing some unwanted bodyweight without having to drastically change your lifestyle.

With this routine, you might actually find yourself having extra time in your hands since you won't be caught up in making plans about where to eat or what to eat. Most people who have adopted Eat Stop Eat lifestyle often find themselves with extra time in their hands. This newly created time is all yours to enjoy and use as you please. You can choose to develop a skill, meditate, reduce your workload, the possibilities are endless.

Positive reinforcement is crucial even as you go through your fasts. Learn to view each completed fast as a small mini-victory towards your ultimate goal of weight loss and a healthy life. This is one of the main differences between traditional dieting and fasting. Dieting gravitates more towards negative reinforcement, where you may go week after week strictly adhering to the diet and then the one day that you eat a cheeseburger seems to have brought down all those weeks of hard work.

With dieting it seems like you are being set up for inevitable failure. A small blunder that you make as you try to diet, teaches your subconscious mind that you will ultimately fail at dieting. However with fasting, each completed fast makes you feel more and more in control of your weight loss plan. It is actually very satisfying to complete a whole day of fasting. Positive reinforcement rather than negative reinforcement is part of what creates sustainability in weight loss.

Why Not Fast For Longer Periods?

24 hours is ideal because it is simple to remember and allows you to at least eat every day. In order to understand why longer fasts are not advisable, we need to understand and appreciate the reciprocal relationship which exists in our bodies between our fat-burning metabolism and our carbohydrate-burning metabolism.

So as to meet the body's energy requirements, your body will burn a blend of fats and carbohydrates. In case you are in the resting state which means you are not participating in any exercises, the "blend" will highly depend on the combination of carbohydrates and fats in your diet. However, as you gradually transition to the fasted state, your metabolism will start to favor fat-burning over carbohydrate-burning. During short fasting periods, your blood sugar levels actually remain stable. Of course, they will drop from the high levels that are experienced after you eat a meal, but they will actually arrive at a stable level which is normally referred to as "fasted level". This fact was discovered by scientist Claude Bernard in 1855. He discovered that during the early stages of fasting, the blood sugar levels were kept stable because of the breakdown of liver glycogen (sugar stored in the liver).

Therefore, liver glycogen is what actually keeps

blood sugar levels stable for short fasting periods. However, if you decide to keep fasting for longer, the liver glycogen will eventually run out and other mechanisms will have to take over so as to maintain the stability of blood sugar levels in the body.

The fasted state metabolism gradually takes over as you extend your fast. The fasted state metabolism is essentially a fat-burning metabolism which maintains your blood sugar levels and preserves the body's protein stores. The longer your fasts are, the more the alterations that must be made to ensure that your body burns as much fat as possible. Basically, the more you extend your fasting period, the more fat burning becomes more dominant than carbohydrate burning. Once you get that far into the fat burning process, you can't just switch it off like a switch by eating a meal. This is where the danger comes in for longer (48 hour or 72 hour) fasts.

An increase in the blood free fatty acids, which result from the breakdown of stored fat, typically forces the muscles to oxidize a large amount of fat into fuel. This leads to the inhibition of glucose oxidation in the muscles. This is a gradual process that starts as early as the 8 to 10 hour mark of the fast and increases as the fast extends and the liver glycogen is slowly depleted.

Fundamentally, it is an established fact that longer fasts (48 to 72 hours and beyond) not only induce an increased level of fat oxidation, but also produce a period of insulin resistance in the muscles during the immediate few hours after breaking the fast. This doesn't happen during 24-hour or shorter fasts since it takes approximately 24 hours to exhaust the liver glycogen.

Therefore, when you fast for longer periods (2 to 3 days and beyond) your body is bound to go into some kind of almost permanent fat burning physiology by down regulating the enzymes and hormones that are responsible for carbohydrate burning. This means that with longer fasts, you will need a longer time to recover once you get back to the fed state because of the insulin resistance that has been generated and the increased hormones and enzymes that were produced. A state of insulin resistance means that even though you are back in the fed state, the body is not responding to the increase of carbohydrates in the body (from eating). This is because it still has to deal with the influx of all the free fatty acids that had been released for a long period of time during the fast. These fatty acids will need time to either be burned off for energy through exercise or stored back as body fat. In addition, the increased growth hormone levels also need time to get back to their normal levels, and this also takes time.

The bottom-line is that with 24-hour or shorter fasts you are able to quickly recover and become more flexible with your fasts. Almost everyone can do a 24-hour fast but not everybody can handle the complications and recovery times of the 48-72 hour or longer fasts. 24-hour fasts once or twice every week that are separated by 2 to 6 days of regular responsible eating and normal exercise routines is a sure way of maintaining overall good health.

"Eat Stop Eat" Style

The purpose of Eat Stop Eat intermittent fasting is not to compel you not to eat but to give you the freedom to eat. Eat Stop Eat actually gives you the freedom to choose when to eat and when not to eat. This is the attitude you should have even as you commit to this style of intermittent fasting. Make sure you are maintaining normal caloric intake even as you maintain your bodyweight. Remember to stick to the golden rule of eating less while you enjoy the foods you eat. Eat plenty of fruits, vegetables, herbs and spices and spend less time worrying about what to eat and what not to eat.

Remember, the aim is to break the destructive cycle

of always being in the fed state. Nutritional experts make the mistake of assuming that you always have to be in the fed state. However, we know that this is not true, since with Eat Stop Eat, we can train our bodies to maintain a balance between the fed and fasted state.

This flawed thinking from the nutritional industry has led to wrong thinking, where all people are obsessed about is what we should eat and what we shouldn't eat. However, there is an angle they are not looking at and it's the angle from which the true solution to sustained long term weight loss and overall health will come from.

With as little as two fasts per week, you are able to create the equivalent of a 20% reduction in calorie intake. For an individual that takes 2,500 calories each day, that is the same as reducing your calorie intake to 2,000 every day. That means your calorie intake has dropped with 500 calories, which is actually the same eliminating a whole cheeseburger and fries from your daily diet. How awesome is that! Even a single fast a week can lead to a 10 % reduction in calorie intake that is sustainable.

Another key thing to remember if you are to commit to Eat Stop Eat is that you require discipline and self-control. This is not a feast and fast method of maintaining good health. After fasting, you just don't go and feast on junk food without a care in the world. You need to at least sustain a maintenance level awareness of what you eat. Basically be responsible with your eating habits but not obsessive about it.

The best approach for you, in case eating a lot makes you gain weight quickly, is to treat your responsible eating habits as weight maintenance as opposed to dieting. Simply watch your bodyweight even as you eat. Remember that all you are doing is breaking from your normal feeding habits; therefore, avoid rituals such as rewarding yourself with large helpings of sugary foods after you end a fast, which you would normally not partake in.

The truth about eating habits is that everyone has their own eating habits based on geographical location, family background, health status and even personal preferences. Therefore, the idea of having one normal or perfect way of eating is a fallacy. Everyone has their own normal feeding habit, therefore there is no "right way of eating", the only rational term that can exist is "responsible eating". Even what we have come to know as common feeding times are different for different people all over the world. For instance in Nepal, breakfast is uncommon and lunch is taken from 9:00 a.m. to 10:00 a.m. In Madrid, lunch is normally taken at 2:00 p.m. while dinner at 9:00 or

10:00 p.m. In Portugal, lunch is around 1:00 p.m. while dinner is around 8:00 p.m. In North America, people eat whenever it's possible; whether standing up, walking to their apartment, in a movie theatre, in a car or on the bed. People eat wherever it's convenient or even sometimes inconvenient.

The problem with most nutritional advice is that it all seems to stem from the idea that the best way to good nutritional habits is avoidance. The problem with human beings is that we naturally do not like rules, the more you are told not to do something, the more you gravitate to doing it. When it comes to dieting, when you are told not to eat a certain food, it becomes even more appealing to you. Therefore, we have more and more people feeling guilty about what they are eating.

Another factor to consider is the "disinhibition" effect, which comes as a result of strict diets. This effect occurs where someone feels so guilty after partaking in food that they had considered off limits that they eventually end up eating even more of it. Generally, the more the foods you have on your bad foods list, the less likely you are to succeed in achieving your goal of losing weight in the long term.

The key to good eating habits is to have a good

relationship with the food you eat. The more you are consciously comfortable with the food you eat, the better off you are. Try as much as possible not to stress about what you eat. The moment you notice you are eating much more than you should, make a conscious decision to stop or plan to compensate for the repercussions in the future.

Attempting to stick to very strict diets is not the solution. This is where Eat Stop Eat comes in as a simple and rational way of dealing with weight loss and establishing sustainable long-term good health. The method may seem somewhat simplistic at first, but it is rational, simple, and flexible. It is applicable no matter where you live in the world.

Another key to good eating habits is variety. Always try to introduce variety in your meals. This way, you will avoid over-partaking or under-partaking in one food nutrient; whether the nutrient is sugar, salt, fat, protein, or any other nutrient. The truth is that even foods that are popularly known as being healthy fade in comparison to meals that have variety. Research has shown that encouraging variety may lead to overeating; this is where self-control comes in. With self- control you are able to eat variety while still keeping your bodyweight in check. Eat Stop Eat provides the perfect platform to practice both variety and self-control and achieve a healthy sustainable balance between the two. Just like the balance advocated for between the fed and fasted state. Eat Stop Eat is more helpful to you when you look at it as a simple, rational, yet potent way to help you eat less. Keep in mind that no one eats perfectly since there is no perfect food or diet. Each and every one of us treat themselves to some dessert or some food that may not be regarded as healthy by most. The only difference is that some feel guilty while others don't. Don't put pressure on yourself to eat in a certain way. All you need to do is learn your eating habits and develop a healthy relationship with your food.

Before You Fast

Always remember to consult your personal physician before making any changes to your diet or beginning any new nutritional program including intermittent fasting. It is important to consult your physician and find out whether this program can be applicable to your individual circumstances. This is especially important in case you are diabetic and on medication.

Remember that nutritional needs usually vary from one person to another, based on age, sex, and health status. In case you are sick, or you generally aren't in good health, it is not advisable to fast.

You can take any non-caloric supplements or vitamins while fasting. However, if you follow the intermittent fasting program properly, you will notice that you don't even need the supplements or vitamins.

Don't worry, you won't lose muscles as long as you eat enough proteins before and after fasts and do some regular resistance exercises. It is perfectly fine to do some light exercises and cardio even while you fast.

A Low Carb High Fat (LCHF) diet goes well with intermittent fasting as it helps the body in fat adaptation. Never use intermittent fasting as an excuse to eat a lot of junk food during your fed state. Try to eat natural, high nutrient foods and avoid processed foods. Also remember to drink plenty of water and non-caloric drinks during your fasts.

In case work gets frantic or you have increased the intensity of your exercises such that fasting is no longer practical for a given period of time, please don't fast. If you do, you may burn out or develop health issues.

Another important thing to consider is the length of your fasting period. You need to decide whether you will be doing a 16-hour, 20-hour or 24-hour fast. Do not overexert yourself. The general rule of thumb in this case is: Do only what is appropriate for you.

The Process of Intermittent Fasting

There are various ways to perform intermittent fasting; however the simplest and most common variations comprise of making use of the natural overnight fasting period by not taking breakfast and simply putting off the first meal of the day by a number of hours. Once you have get passed the 12-hour mark from the dinner that you had the previous night, you are actually in a fasted state and you start to depend on stored body fat for energy.

Keep in mind that the longer you remain in this fasted state, the more metabolic training your body will get of burning stored fat and the better your body's fat adaptation will get. In fact, if you are able to sustain this fast for 20 to 24 hours, you will be able to reach a very high level of lipolysis (breakdown of stored fat into free fatty acids, which can then be used as fuel in the cells) and fat oxidation (the burning of fat in mitochondria found in the cells).

During your first experience with intermittent fasting, you may experience hunger, low energy levels and other symptoms. That is why it is recommended that you start with "baby steps", don't overexert yourself. You can start by just pushing breakfast out by an hour or two, then gradually and continuously increasing the fasting period. With time, your body will become more "fat adapted", and it will eventually become easier to fast for longer intervals. It is actually similar to physical exercise whereby those who are used to a sedentary lifestyle find it hard and even painful at first, but with time their bodies and minds adapt and it starts becoming easier and enjoyable.

Low Carb High Fat Diet (LCHF) for Fat Adaptation

In case you are going to diet while you fast, it is much simpler to fast if you are on a LCHF diet. This is because LCHF foods naturally result in quite a bit of fat adaptation and lead to lesser secretion of insulin and use of glucose as fuel. The combination of a LCHF diet with intermittent fasting is actually recommended. The closer you are to a ketogenic diet (extremely low in carbs, moderate in proteins, and rich in fat diet - encouraging the production of keytone bodies) the simpler it will be for you to go for more hours without feeding, because of the fat adaptation that such diets create.

For those who choose to include carbohydrates in their diet, it is recommended that it mostly consists of fibre (non- digestible carbs), which essentially should not result in the increase of glucose and insulin. If by any chance you then decide to take digestible carbs (which is not recommended) you should avoid eating them early in the day, since it will sabotage the fat-burning process, and set you up for food cravings throughout the day.

If you really have to eat non-fiber carbs, ensure you take them in the evening, after a long period of fasting or after an intense physical exercise session. This is so as to ensure that the liver and muscle glycogen have been depleted; otherwise your whole fasting period would have been counter-productive.

Remember, do not fast if you are sick or you have

committed to doing long and strenuous exercises.

Intermittent fasting is a flexible and long-term solution, one week you may choose to fast once a week, the next week twice, just do what is appropriate for you!

Special Considerations For Fasting Women

It is no surprise that there are gender differences when it comes to how our human bodies function. Men and women have different appearance, metabolism and physiology. Actually, there are many books that have been written about this topic. One good book you could check out is Dr. Mark Tarnopolsky's "Gender Differences in Metabolism". Men and women differ in terms of body fat levels and muscle mass. Additionally, women have different physiological and metabolic needs that relate to their unique child bearing physiology. This is a fact that simply cannot be overlooked when we are discussing about weight loss strategies such as dieting and fasting. Therefore, it would be fitting for us to look at fasting and women as a special consideration.

Generally, women have the tendency to burn more fat than men on a day-to-day basis and are more sensitive to insulin than men. To start with, there are the obvious hormonal differences like estrogen and testosterone which actually affect the ability of the human body to burn fat and form muscle. These hormones also have an influence on where body fat will be stored.

Women have a more diverse and unique hormonal profile compared to men. There are huge differences between men and women in fat loss hormones. Generally, men have less growth hormones circulating in their bodies than women. Women also have two to three times more leptin compared to men. Men's hormone levels are more stable than women's, since women's hormone levels fluctuate within their menstrual cycles.

High estrogen levels increase blood growth hormone and leptin levels; this is a fact that was proved by a study conducted on premenopausal versus post-menopausal women. A combination of elevated estrogen levels and elevated growth hormone levels is one of the indicators of a healthy woman. A healthy young woman is capable of producing twice or even seven times as much growth hormone than men, prepubescent girls or post-menopausal women.

Due to the above mentioned hormonal differences, women will have more free fatty acids released into their blood stream after longer fasts of around 40 to 72 hours. This means that a woman will linger more in the fat burning metabolic state than a man after a long fast. This fact is evidenced by the fact that immediately after breaking the fast, there will be elevated fat oxidation levels even after meals, and slow glucose clearance. There will also be a relative inability of increased insulin to reduce the fat burning process and increase the carb-burning process. Since we have established that it is true that women have a unique physiology that affects their fat burning process, how then does this fact affect their ability to lose weight? First and foremost, it is a well-known fact that huge energy deficits may cause menstrual dysfunction in women. These energy deficits may be caused by long periods of food deficiency, intense exercise sessions and hurried weight loss strategies. This is a phenomenon that is often witnessed in women who choose to diet for prolonged periods and female athletes who fail to meet the caloric threshold for their rigorous training routines.

It is not just huge amounts of caloric deficits over long periods that can be a problem. Even extremely low levels of body fat can be a problem for women. Frisch and McArthur in 1974 developed the theory that a 22%-body fat level is critical to the preservation of normal menstrual functions. The research of Frisch and McArthur points to the importance of having fat in the body, though the critical level should be more of a percentage range. This goes for all human beings, the goal of fasting is not to achieve zero percent body fat but to burn off unhealthy body fat. Nothing good can come from having extremely low body fat.

For men, the critical body fat level ranges between 4 to 6%, it may vary based on ethnicity or age. Men's critical level is actually below half of that of women. However, as human beings we all need fat in order for our bodies to function properly. Otherwise we may develop metabolic or hormonal issues.

A study that was conducted on elite female athletes indicated that a combination of decreased body fat levels and a huge calorie deficit in the female body may lead to amenorrhea (an unusual absence of a woman's menstrual periods) in addition to low estradiol and leptin levels.

In this particular study, it was discovered that the more trim female athletes were the once that tended to have amenorrhea, had decreased insulin, estradiol and leptin. Most of these athletes were approximately 23 years of age, had a Body Mass Index (BMI) of roughly 18 and body fat levels of approximately 15%.

For instance, a 5 foot 6 inch tall woman in this study would possibly have the weight of approximately 112 pounds; they would most likely burn roughly 1,000 calories every day through workout, all while eating about 1,700 calories and around 55 grams of protein each day.

For those female athletes that still had normal menstruation, it was discovered that they had a bit more body fat (approximately 15.5%), they had nearly the exact amount of lean mass as their counterparts who had amenorrhea , however they ate around 500 more calories per day, and considerably more protein (78 grams a day). They were found to have higher levels of insulin, leptin, thyroid hormones than their counterparts.

Although this is not a scenario where these women were fasting, the study indicates that low body fat combined with prolonged calorie deficit and slight protein deficit can cause significant hormonal disruptions.

There are definitely hormonal and physiological differences between men and women as illustrated above. However, this does not mean that either men or women cannot participate in intermittent fasting. Each gender has their own unique hurdles which they may face in case they want to reap the benefits of fasting.

Women are generally immune to the stress that comes with 72 hour fasts compared to men. A study was carried out on a group of men and women who had fasted for 4 consecutive days; it was later found that they all experienced a drop in the active form of thyroid hormone (T3). However there was a greater drop in the men than the women. This was not due to body weight or weight loss differences but due to the hormonal differences between men and women.

It has also been discovered that women tend to recover their sensitivity to insulin faster than men during shorter fasts of around 12 to 38 hours. However, their sensitivity to insulin becomes worse for prolonged fasts such as 48 to 72 hour fasts, this is because they release more free fatty acids compared to men.

Another interesting difference is that men's testosterone levels tend to decrease during prolonged fasts and although women's testosterone level is significantly lower than that of men, it does not change during the fast. Women also have more fat burning enzymes compared to men, therefore are able to burn more fat. Even when a man and a woman are matched in terms of fat mass, the woman will release and burn more body fat than the man during periods of calorie deprivation.

Women are more suited for short fasts because of their ability to release more free fatty acids in the blood, their ability to burn more fat faster, their increased level of growth hormones and their low vulnerability to metabolic disruptions. When women commit to different forms of intermittent fasting, they experience improved health benefits such as burning off of excess visceral fat. They also experience improved sensitivity to insulin and improved levels of cholesterol and triglyceride.

Extremely lean or overly active women are more limited when it comes to fasting variety, as we shall see. An experiment was carried out to analyze the effect that fasting has on women who are very lean. In this experiment, 8 extremely lean and healthy women who had a BMI of approximately 20 or less and body fat of 20% or less took part in a fasting period of 72 hours while they were in the mid-follicular stage (important phase of follicular development) of their monthly cycle.

A classic woman in this experiment would have the following characteristics: 28 years of age, 5 feet 6 inches in height, 120 pounds in weight and about 19% body fat. This level of body fat is very close to the 12% "essential" level that is quoted as the minimal for women by the American Council on Exercise. This means that the ladies involved in this study were already exceptionally lean.

All the ladies who participated in the experiment were actively involved in exercises, with one of them involved in exercise for longer than 1.5 hours every day for 5 days in a week(very remarkable). The exercises included: weight lifting, cycling, walking and aerobic dancing. The hypothesis of the researchers was that, it would be extremely difficult to find that all these 8 ladies were having normal monthly cycles after the fasting period.

After the fast, the typical woman in the experiment had lost 5 pounds, leading to the weight of the typical 5 feet 6 inches woman moving down to 115 pounds. This leads to the BMI dropping to approximately 18 to 19.

Other changes that accompanied the drop in weight included increase in cortisol levels and late development of the follicles. During the experiment, one of the ladies experienced amenorrhea.

The findings stated above were found to be directly contrasting an almost similar experiment that was carried out by the same scientists. This other experiment was carried out on a group of ladies that had 25% body fat. In the experiment, 12 ladies who were close to their ideal bodyweight by 15% were observed as they undertook a 72-hour fast. This was done while in they were in the mid-follicular stage of their monthly cycle; same as in the other experiment with the lean women.

In this particular experiment follicular development was observed through estradiol measurements and ultrasound examinations on a daily basis. The findings indicated that follicle development was the same in all the cycles and was succeeded by ovulation in all the ladies involved. The follicular and luteal stage durations of both the fed and fasted cycles were also the same. Therefore, 72 hour fasts seemed to have relatively lesser effect on the reproductive physiology of women with normal bodyweight. If you compare the two experiments, for the lean women and the women with normal bodyweight, a clear conclusion can be drawn out. The conclusion is that lean women run a higher risk of developing follicular and neuroendocrine reproductive complications during prolonged fasting periods (72 hours).

The fact is that based on research, 72 hours fasts are too lengthy for ladies who are already exceptionally lean and active physically. These fasts may even prove to be detrimental to the reproductive cycles of lean women.

Even though women may seem to be generally incompatible with longer fasts, it is not necessarily so. Men also experience a considerable decrease in testosterone during 72 hour fasting periods. Therefore the reproductive effects of long caloric deficits are similar to both men and women although they are more conspicuous for women. Generally, longer fasts have detrimental results for both lean and active men and women. This is the same case with anyone from either gender who combines strict dieting or intense physical exercise with fasting. You may end up burning out or binge eating after your fasts.

Estrogen levels are another trait that is unique to women. Studies in both animals and humans have shown that the ingestion of food fluctuates in various stages of menstruation. For instance, it is low in the pre-ovulatory stage and high in the initial follicular and luteal stages. Estrogen tends to depress the appetite, through lowering the body's sensitivity to food indicators such as smell. Therefore, depending on its prevalence in the body, women may find it easier of harder to diet or fast depending on the phase of the menstrual cycle that they are in.

As we have seen, there are significant differences in how men and women react to fasting or dieting. Through the research that we have looked at, there are no factual indicators that advocate that either gender should not participate in fasting. There are also no indicators that either of the genders can fast carelessly as much as they want without being rational.

Fasting must be done rationally and wisely. 24-hour fasts are adequate for you to experience significant weight loss results for both genders. Although there is the temptation to prolong your fasts for faster and better results, remember, there is such a thing as "too much of a good thing".

Ideally, 24-hour fasts are meant to be a replacement

for traditional dieting and extreme exercises, as you journey towards your weight loss goal. However, minor dietary inclusions such as a Low Carb High Fat diet can be incorporated with moderation.

Just like with exercise or dieting, fasting can be overdone. Prolonging your fasts may end up having counterproductive results as we have seen. The key to intermittent fasting as a solution to weight loss is fitting it naturally into your life and allowing yourself time to loss that unwanted bodyweight at a natural and sustainable pace.

As a wise man once said, "patience is the key". Don't try to force weight loss because it will backfire on you. Always remember, attaining zero percent body fat is not the goal of intermittent fasting; losing unwanted bodyweight and maintaining your weight loss through living a healthy lifestyle should be your ultimate goal, whether you are a man or woman.

Key Things To Remember

The key to intermittent fasting is to teach your body to get used to taking a break from eating, and break the habit of always being in the fed state. Liquids are very important during your fasts. Calorie-free beverages and calorie-free gums (in moderation) are okay to take during your fasts. However, avoid any other foods even though they may have small amounts of calories. Eating responsibly is a mindset. You will always find yourself at some point in your life where you want to eat more, even though it might be detrimental to your health. Remember, there is no good thing that comes easy. Commit to eating sensibly, you just can't devour all you want and still lose weight. Even getting your body fat surgically removed won't be a long term solution. As long as your attitude towards food does not change, you will always end up filling those spaces that were surgically removed.

The key to responsible eating is developing a healthy relationship with food. Spend less time worrying about what to eat and remember that if you can do without a certain unhealthy food, then exclude it. However, if you absolutely can't do without it, then don't. Introduce variety in your meals.

The secret to fasting intermittently is rational simplicity. It may seem over-simplistic but it is the best way to achieve sustainable long term weight loss. Basically, enjoy the food you eat, introduce nutritional diversity in what you eat and remember to take non-caloric liquids during your fasts. Always do what works for you; that is the key to sustainability. Don't try to copy what a friend who is getting results is doing. Learn your eating habits, start fasting slowly and work your way up. Don't try to force weight loss by combining strict dieting, fasting and extreme exercise routines in order to achieve fast results. Be patient and allow yourself to lose weight at a natural pace. Recurring fasting is an effective technique to consuming that is coming to be preferred since it could help you reduce weight without really feeling cravings, and also help in reducing your threat of persistent conditions like diabetic issues as well as cardiovascular disease. Periodic fasting could additionally lead to much better rest and also whole lots of energy if done appropriately. Chronic Fatigue Syndrome may vanish forever.

* * *

Throughout history, fasting is a widespread technique,

which has been a spiritual practice for centuries. Today, contemporary science has actually verified that fasting returns the list below perks:

* Aids market of the hormone insulin level of "sensitivity" - Optimizing the hormone insulin level is important for you health and wellness, as the hormone insulin resistance, or the hormone insulin level of sensitivity, adds to almost ALL persistent illness
* Stabilizes Gherkin Degrees, also called you "cravings for bodily hormones". IF boosts high levels of HGH, which plays an important role in your overall health and wellness, and in slowing down the aging process!
* Decreases Triglycerides * Assists in reducing swelling and inflammation, thereby easing the pain of arthritis and gout. Furthermore, working out in a fasted state could aid to neutralize muscular tissue, as well as enhance fat burning.

Eat Stop Eat has been popularized by the bodybuilder Brad Pilon. It comprises of fasting for a whole 24 hour period, once or twice per week. This method is quite tasking and is only recommended for a maximum of two non-consecutive times per week.

With this method you are guaranteed an extremely deep level of fat adaptation and very low levels of insulin. Some people think that this might cause them to eat too much food the following day, however this is not true. Studies have shown that even though you might eat very much the next day, you will not even come close to the amount you would have taken for both days if you weren't fasting. With this protocol, each day you successfully fast gives you 12 hours of fasting above the baseline. This means that two fasts a week give you 24 hours (a day) of fasting.

Bottom-line

With each of these fasting methods, you are basically skipping breakfast, avoiding snacking during the fasting periods and consolidating your calorie intake as you near the end of the day. All of these methods are effective and you can actually choose to mix and match.

Remember to keep it flexible, any fasting beyond 12

hours is actually beneficial. Don't sweat it if you can't achieve your target for the day, as long as you have fasted, you are better off than if you had eaten all day long.

A good goal to have would be a 24-hour weekly aggregate of extra fasting above the baseline. This would mean: 2 days of Eat Stop Eat or 3 days of the Warrior Diet or 6 days of Lean-gains fasting method. You are free to mix and match based on your lifestyle, preferences, schedule or level of fat adaptation.

Non-caloric drinks

During your fasts you are free to take non-caloric drinks such as water, black coffee, black tea, non-caloric diet soda. Avoid putting cream in your coffee. However, if you absolutely must take cream, don't stop fasting because you can't do without cream or sugar.

Try and get used to black coffee or tea as you breakfast as you fast. You will find that you will spend less time worrying about what you will take for breakfast and be able to concentrate on what is really important. Research has also shown that you are more focused or alert in your fasted state. Black coffee and tea also contain compounds that assist with the breaking down of fats and have a bunch of other health benefits.

Eat Stop Eat Intermittent Fasting

Let's take an in-depth look at Eat Stop Eat intermittent fasting since it is the most flexible and comprehensive of all the methods that have been highlighted above. With the Eat Stop Eat Plan, a 24-hour period of intermittent fasting is recommended. However as you will soon see, even shorter periods of fasting can work with the Eat Stop Eat Plan.

Let's say you want to fast for 24 hours, all you need to do is eat as you normally would until 6:00 pm on the first day, and then fast until 6:00 pm on day two. For instance, you could start your fast on Sunday at 6:00 pm and end it on Monday at 6:00 pm. This fasting strategy is sometimes referred to as the dinner-to-dinner fast, because of the fasting timeframe.

Through following this plan you are able to eat every day while at the same time, take a break from eating for 24 hours. This ensures that you are able to reset the metabolic balance between the fed and fasted state. Therefore you are not continuously in the fed or fasted state.

Remember that the timeframe of 6:00 pm to 6:00 pm is not set in stone and can be changed to suite your lifestyle or personal preference. In case a dinner-to-dinner fast is not appropriate for you, you can try a different timeframe, such as, 2:00 pm to 2:00 pm, which may be referred to as a lunch-to-lunch fast.

Intermittent fasting in this plan is very flexible. The key thing to aim for is to be asleep during the periods in the fast that you find the hardest. For instance, in case you find the start of a fast tougher than the end, you may consider fasting between 8 pm and 8 pm. In this case, you may be asleep by 9 or 10 pm, which basically means you won't have to struggle through the beginning hours of your fast. The flexibility of intermittent fasting also extends to the days. Let's say you had planned to start a dinner-to-dinner fast on Wednesday, however something came up. For instance, your friends invited you for a celebration dinner since one of them got promoted. You don't need to worry; you can simply put off the fast to the next day or another different day. Remember, as long as you are fasting once or twice a week, you are still working within the plan.

The beauty of intermittent fasting is that it can change with the way your life is changing. For instance, dinner-to- dinner fasts may be working for you when you start; however as time goes by, you may find that it is getting harder and harder to finish your fasts or that you are getting a strong urge to overeat after your fasts. In such a case, you could switch to a different fasting timeframe.

You will notice that shifting from one fasting timeframe to another may yield better and more consistent results, depending on your lifestyle. It is advisable to switch through different timeframes and try them out before extending the duration of your fasts so as to ensure that you are working with the best timeframe for your needs. Unlike dieting where you can only eat specific foods and have to adhere to a strict dietary plan, intermittent fasting works better with flexibility. The truth is that flexibility is the key to sustainable long-term weight loss.

Water is still very important even as you fast. With intermittent fasting you can drink calorie-free beverages of your choice. Below is a list of some of the drinks that are permissible during the fasting period:

• Black tea • Black Coffee • Herbal tea • Green tea • Water • Diet soda pop • Sparkling water

Remember that a significant share of your daily liquid intake is gotten from the food you take. Therefore, since you are not taking any food during the fasting period, it is important to take more drinks than normal in order to compensate for the liquid that could have been gotten from the normal food intake.

It is important to try your best to keep you calorie

intake as close to zero as possible during your fast. If you try adding a little bit of sugar or cream to your drink, it is inevitable that your calorie intake will start to rise during your fasting period. Try your best to have zero tolerance towards calorie-intake during your fasts, in order to achieve the best results from your fasts.

I know some of you might be thinking: "what about foods that are low in calories, can we take a small portion of these during our fasts?" These kinds of foods may include but are not limited to the following: beef broth, coconut water, or xylitol. Currently, the research that is available is not enough to answer questions on the metabolic effect of small quantities of calories from various foods and ingredient sources.

The genuine answer to the question asked above would be – the key to intermittent fasting is taking a complete break from eating food for a predetermined period of time, please don't try to game the system. Just stick to the basics; otherwise this would become a dietary plan. In order to achieve the best results, just stick to the basics of keeping off food completely during your fast and resume eating after the fast, simple enough.

However, we are not ignorant of the fact that some of you may not be able to keep off certain foods because of health reasons. Therefore the general rule about what you can or cannot eat during your fast, would be – "*If you can go without then go without, but if you really can't go without then don't.*

Flexibility of Eat Stop Eat Intermittent Fasting

To start off, try one fast per week. During this time, you can experiment what timeframe works best for you. After you get used to fasting and zero in on an appropriate timeframe, you can then increase the number of fasts per week.

Avoid the mistake of trying to fit in as many fasts as you can in a week or trying to extend a fast for more than 24 hours, in a bid to get faster results. Extending beyond the 24-hour recommended period reduces the flexibility of intermittent fasting and may lead to a fasting burnout. If you do this, you will find yourself dreading the next fasting period, which essentially defeats the whole point of fasting. Just like with physical exercises where you require recovery time so as to enable your muscles to build, so is the case with fasting. The benefits of fasting do not end with the fasted state but also extend to the fed state, where you get more energy to go through the next fasted state. A 48-hour recovery period is recommended between two 24-hour fasting periods. Essentially what you are doing is getting your body to get used to this cycle of moving from a fed state to a fasted state instead of continuously being in the fed state. Remember, we are not trying to move completely to the fasted state either; we are trying to achieve a metabolic balance between the two.

Research has shown that those people, who stay flexible and relaxed during intermittent fasting, achieve the best weight loss results and are also able to keep the weight off after losing it. On the other hand, those people who try to speed up the process through extending their fasts to 48 hours or 72 hours actually see quick results but are more likely to have severe weight rebounds once they break one of their fasting rules.

This is because those people who overexert themselves are more likely to burn out quicker than those who take their time to understand what works for them and are open to being more flexible with their fasts. Generally, the more rules you try to follow in nutrition (bad food/good food lists, good food combinations/bad food combinations, etc.) the more likely you will see quick weight loss results. However, the more the rules, the more likely you will experience punishing weight rebounds in case you break some of your rules and restraints. Similarly with intermittent fasting, if you have restrained fasting periods, you will find yourself feeling guilty if you overeat or break a fast. This would not be the case if you had flexible fasting periods. The purpose of intermittent fasting is to stop obsessive compulsive eating and move to a healthy metabolic balance between the fed and fasted state. You should not move to the other extreme of obsessing about fasting.

It is also not advisable to combine fasting and strict dieting plans or extreme exercises. This may lead to a burnout. The best indicator to show you that you are not approaching weight loss properly is if you are straining to organize fasting, exercising and dieting within the same schedule. In this case, you are doing too much of one activity. Fasting and light but strenuous exercise is a good combination when properly planned within a schedule.

With intermittent fasting, you can do weight training at least twice per week. If you wish, you can add cardio exercises, but remember to recover adequately from your fasts and workouts. Essentially, your once or twice a week fasts are supposed to replace your traditional dieting. Nonetheless, if you have a significant amount of weight to lose then you can fast and at the same time eat with a slight deficit during your fed state. As a general rule of thumb, in case you are fasting, while in your fed state (on the days you are eating) you should not experience more than a 10 to 20% food deficit in your body for any length of time. The leaner you become, the less likely you need to combine dieting and fasting. It is important to keep in mind that the goal is not to achieve 0% body fat. With fasting, you are losing weight simply by doing nothing and therefore there is no need to complicate things any further through dieting. Remember, every completed fast is a milestone towards achieving your goal; therefore you should celebrate and reward yourself by enjoying what you eat.

Conclusion

I have personally been a student of IF for many years now. I can attest to the benefits from this practice. I honestly believe, without a shadow of doubt, that if you implement what has been explained here in this short book, you will begin to see changes in your body and mind that you never thought possible. You will regain a feeling of self-worth, and you will become healthier.

Please don't take my word for it. Try this "new way" of eating, and see for yourself! I whole-heartedly appreciate you purchasing my book and reading through the pages. But, I gain nothing if you don't act now by consulting with our physician, and beginning this awesome, life-changing regimen! My sincere thanks.

If you are interested in more information about IF, I would suggest you try a system created by Brad Pilon. Brad is an internationally recognized intermittent fasting advocate and author of Eat Stop Eat. In the system, Brad shares a very simple weight loss strategy for men and women who want to experience fat loss without dieting, or changing the foods they eat. His system is proven to help you lose weight without losing muscle and/or energy!

Basically, Brad will take you further in your journey to lose weight and get healthy. His system has been proven to work countless times for thousands of people. I am personally a student of Brad's, and I would like to acknowledge him as a true guru when it comes to Intermittent Fasting!

My sincere thanks! Faron T Connelly

"Looking good and feeling good go hand in hand. If you have a healthy lifestyle, your diet and nutrition are set, and you're working out, you're going to feel good".
Jason Statham"

Acknowledgements

"Eat Stop Eat" References The following references were obtained and provided to you here, in an effort to help you with educating yourself further about intermittent fasting. 1 Swinburn B, Sacks G, Ravussin E. Increased food energy supply is more than sufficient to explains the US epidemic of obesity. Am J Clin Nutr 2009; 90:1453-6 2 Li C, Ford ES, Zhao G, Balluz LS, Giles WH. Estimates of body composition with dual-energy X-ray absorptiometry in adults. Am J Clin Nutr. 2009; 90(6):1457-65 3 Adams KM, Kohlmeier M, Zeisel SH. Nutrition Education in U.S. Medical Schools: LatestUpdate of a National Survey. Academic Medicine. 2010; 85(9): 1537- 1542 4 Marion Nestle. Eating Made Simple. Scientific American Magazine, September 2007. 5 Marion Nestle. What to Eat. New York, New York: North Point Press 2006 (For more information visit www.whattoeatbook.com) 6 University of Guelph, Unpublished Research, in Review. 7 Marion Nestle. Food politics. Los Angeles, California: University of California Press. 2003

8 Brian Wansink. Marketing Food. Cha0mpaign, Illinois: University of Illinois Press. 2005 9 Paul Campos. The Obesity Myth. New York, New York: Gotham Books.

2004

10 Cuneen SA. Review of meta-analytic comparisons of bariatric surgery with a focus on laparoscopic adjustable gastric banding. Surgery for Obesity and Related Diseases. 2008;4: S47-S55.

11 Buchwald H, Avidor Y, Braunwald E, et al. Bariatric surgery a systematic review and meta-analysis. Journal of the American Medical Association. 2004; 292:1724-37. 12 Webber J, Macdonald IA. The cardiovascular, metabolic and hormonal changes accompanying acute starvation in men and women. British Journal of Nutrition. 1994; 71:437-447.

13 Heilbronn LK, et al. Alternate-day fasting in non-obese subjects: effects on body weight, body composition, and energy metabolism. American Journal of Clinical Nutrition. 2005; 81:69-73

14 Keim NL, Horn WF. Restrained eating behavior and the metabolic response to dietary energy restriction in women. Obesity Research. 2004; 12:141-149. 15 Verboeket-Van De Venne WPHG, et al. Effect of the pattern of food intake on human energy metabolism. British Journal of Nutrition. 1993; 70:103-115

16 Bellisle F, et al. Meal Frequency and energy balance. British Journal of Nutrition. 1997; 77: (Suppl. 1)

s57-s70 17 Gjedsted J, et al. Effects of a 3-day fast on regional lipid and glucose metabolism in human skeletal muscle and adipose tissue. Acta Physiologica Scandinavia 207; 191:205-216

18 Gardner CD, et al. Comparison of the Atkins, Zone, Ornish, and LEARN diets on change in weight and related risk factors among overweight premenopausal women. The A to Z weight loss study: A randomized trial. Journal of the American Medical Association. 2007; 297(9): 969-998

Eat Stop Eat 190 19 Hultman E. Physiological role of muscle glycogen in man, with special reference to exercise. Circ Res 1967;20(suppl 1):199-114 20 Knapik JJ, Jones BH, Meredith C, Evans WJ. Influence of a 3.5 day fast on physical performance. European Journal of Applied Physiology and Occupational Physiology 1987; 56(4):428-32 21 Schisler JA, Ianuzzo CD. Running to maintain cardiovascular fitness is not limited by short-term fasting or enhanced by carbohydrate supplementation. Journal of Physical Activity and Health. 2007 Jan;4(1):101- 12. 22 Knapik JJ, Meredith CN, Jones LS, Young VR, Evans WJ. Influence of fasting on carbohydrate and fat metabolism during rest and exercise in men. Journal of Applied Physiology 1998; 64(5): 1923-1929 23 Nieman

DC, et al. Running endurance in 27-h-fasted humans. Journal of Applied Physiology 1987; 63(6):2502- 2509

24 Zinker BA, Britz K, Brooks GA. Effects of a 36-hour fast on human endurance and substrate utilization. Journal Applied Physiology 1990; 69(5): 1849-1855 25 Aragon-Vargas LF. Effects of fasting on endurance exercise. Sports Med 1993; 16:255-65

26 Gleeseon M, Greenhaff PL, Maughan RJ. Influence of a 24 h fast on a high intensity cycle exercise performance in man. Eur J Appl Physiol Occup Physiol 1988;46:211-19 27 Dohm, GL, Beeker RT, Isreal RG, Tapscott EB. Metabolic responses to exercise after fasting. Journal of Applied Physiology 61(4): 1363-1368,1986.

28 Hermansen L, Vaage O. Lactate disappearance and glycogen synthesis in human muscle after maximal exercise. Am J Phsiol 1977; 233:E422-9. 29 Muthayya S, Thomas T, Srinivasan K, Rao K, Kurpad AV, van Klinken JW, Owen G, de Bruin EA. Consumption of a mid-morning snack improves memory but not attention in school children. Physiology & Behavior. 2007 Jan 30;90(1):142-50.

30 Green MW, Elliman NA, Rogers, PJ. Lack of effect of short-term fasting on cognitive function. Journal of Psychiatric Research 1995; 29(3), 245-253. 31

Leiberman HR, Caruso CM, Niro PJ, Adam GE, Kellogg MD, Nindl B, Kramer FM. A double-blind, placebo-controlled test of 2 d of calorie deprivation: effects on cognition, activity, sleep, and interstitial glucose concentrations. American Journal of Clinical Nutrition 2008;88:667–76.

32 Green MW, Rogers PJ, Elliman NA, Gatenby SJ. Impairment of cognitive performance associated with dieting and high levels of dietary restraint. Physiology and Behavior. 1994;55(3):447-52.

33 Green MW, Rogers PJ. Impaired cognitive functioning during spontaneous dieting. Psychological Medicine. 1995;25(5):1003-10. 34 Witte AV, Fobker M, Gellner R, Knecht S, Flöel A. Caloric restriction improves memory in elderly humans. The Proceedings of the National Academy of Sciences. 2009 Jan 27;106(4):1255-60

35 Bryner RW. Effects of resistance training vs. Aerobic training combined with an 800 calorie liquid diet on lean body mass and resting metabolic rate. Journal of the American College of Nutrition 1999; 18(1): 115- 121

Eat Stop Eat 191

36 Rice B, Janssen I, Hudson, R, Ross R. Effects of aerobic or resistance exercise and/or diet on glucose

tolerance and plasma insulin levels in obese men. Diabetes Care 1999; 22: 684-691

37 Janssen I, et al. Effects of an energy-restrictive diet with or without exercise on abdominal fat, intermuscular fat, and metabolic risk factors in obese women. Diabetes Care 2002; 25:431-438

38 Chomentowski P, et al. Moderate Exercise Attenuates the Loss of Skeletal MuscleMass That Occurs With Intentional Caloric Restriction – Induced Weight Loss in Older, Overweight to Obese Adults. Journal of Gerontology: MEDICAL SCIENCES. 2009. Vol. 64A, No. 5, 575–580

39 Marks BL, Ward A, Morris DH, Castellani J, and Rippe RM. Fat-free mass is maintained in women following a moderate diet and exercise program. Medicine and Science in Sports and Exercise. 1995; 27(9): 1243-51

40 Gjedsted J, Gormsen L, Buhl M, Norrelund H, Schmitz, Keiding S, Tonnesen E, Moller N. Forearm and leg amino acids metabolism in the basal state and during combined insulin and amino acid stimulation after a 3- day fast. Acta Physiologica. 2009; (6): 1-9.

41 Gibala MJ, Interisano SA, Tarnopolsky MA et al. (2000) Myofibrillar disruption following acute concentric and

eccentric resistance exercise in strength-trained men. Can J Physiol Pharmacol 78, 656–661 42 Bray GA, Smith SR, De Jonge L, Xie H, Rood J, Martin CK, Most M, Brock C, Manscuso S, Redman LM.

Effect of Dietary Protein Content on Weight Gain, Energy Expenditure, and Body Composition During Overeating. JAMA. 2012;307(1):47-55 43 Deldicque L, De Bock K, Maris M, Ramaekers M, Nielens H, Francaux M, Hespel P. Increased p70s6k phosphorylation during intake of a protein-carbohydrate drink following resistance exercise in the fasted state. Eur J Appl Physiol. 2010 Mar;108(4):791-800.

44 Samer W. El-Kadi, Agus Suryawan, Maria C. Gazzaneo, Neeraj Srivastava, Renán A. Orellana, Hanh V. Nguyen, Gerald E. Lobley, and Teresa A. Davis. Anabolic signaling and protein deposition are enhanced by intermittent compared with continuous feeding in skeletal muscle of neonates. Am J Physiol Endocrinol Metab 2012;302 E674-E686

45 Van Proeyen K, De Bock K, Hespel P. Training in the fasted state facilitates re-activation of eEF2 activity during recovery from endurance exercise. Eur J Appl Physiol. 2011 Jul;111(7):1297-305.

46 Phillips SM, Tipton KD, Aarsland A et al. (1997)

Mixed muscle protein synthesis and breakdown after resistance exercise in humans. Am J Physiol 273(1 Pt 1), E99–107. 47 Rasmussen BB, Tipton KD, Miller SL, Wolf SE, Wolfe RR. An oral essential amino acid-carbohydrate supplement enhances muscle protein anabolism after resistance exercise. J Appl Physiol. 2000:88;386-392.

48 Tipton KD, Rasmussen BB, Miller SL, Wolf SE, Owens-Stovall SK, Petrini BE, Wolfe RR. Timing of amino acid-carbohydrate ingestion alters anabolic response of muscle to resistance exercise. Am J Physiol Endocrinol Metab. 2001 Aug;281(2):E197-206.

49 Burd NA, West DW, Moore DR, Atherton PJ, Staples AW, Prior T, Tang JE, Rennie MJ, Baker SK, Phillips SM. Enhanced amino acid sensitivity of myofibrillar protein synthesis persists for up to 24 h after resistance exercise in young men. J Nutr. 2011 Apr 1;141(4):568-73.

50 Phillips SM, Tipton KD, Aarsland A, Wolf SE, Wolfe RR. Mixed muscle protein synthesis and breakdown Eat Stop Eat 192 after resistance exercise in humans. Am J Physiol 1997;273(36):E99-E107

51 Brian Wansink. Mindless Eating. New York, New York: Bantam Dell (A division of Random House, Inc.) 2006

52 Agatson, Arthur. The South Beach Diet. New York, New York: Rodale Inc. 2003 53Grimm O. Addicted to food. Scientific American Mind 2007; 18(2):36-39 54 Ozelli KL (Interviewing Volkow ND). This is your brain on food. Scientific American Magazine. September, 2007.

55 Rogers PJ, Smith HJ. Food cravings and food "addiction": a critical review of the evidence from a biopsychosocial perspective. Pharmacology biochemistry and Behavior 2000;66(1): 3-14

56 Lowe MR, Butryn ML. Hedonic hunger: a new dimension of appetite? Physiol Behav 2007; 91: 432–439. 57 Honma KL, Honma S, Hiroshige T. Critical role of food amount for prefeeding cortcosterone peak in rats. American Journal of Physiology. 1983; 245: R339-R344. 58Comperatore CA, Stephan FK. Entrainment of duodenal activity to periodic feeding. Journal of Biological Rhythms. 1987; 2:227-242.

59 Stephan FK. The "other" circadian system" food as a Zeitgeber Journal of Biological Rhythms. 2002; 17:284- 292. 60 Steffens AB, 1976 Influence of the oral cavity on insulin release in the rat AM J PHysiol 230:1411-1415

61 Johnstone AM, Faber P, Gibney ER, Elia M, Horgan G, Golden BE, Stubbs RJ. Effect of an acute fast on

energy

compensation and feeding behaviour in lean men and women. Int J Obes Relat Metab Disord. 2002 Dec;26(12):1623-8. 62 Guettier JM, Gorden P. Hypoglycemia. Endocrinology Clinics of North America. 2006; 35:753–766

63 Wiesli P, Schwegler B, Schmid B, Spinas GA, Schmid C. Mini-mental state examination is superior to plasma glucose concentrations in monitoring patients with suspected hypoglycemic disorders during the 72-hour fast. European Journal of Endocrinololgy 2005;152: 605–610. 64 Alken J, et al. Effect of fasting on young adults who have symptoms of hypoglycemia in the absence of frequent meals. European Journal of Clinical Nutrition 2008; 62: 721–726

65 Halaas J, Gajiwala K, Maffei M, Cohen S, Chait B, et al. Weight-reducing effects of the plasma protein encoded by the obese gene. Science 1995; 269:543–46 66 Chan JL, et al. Short-term fasting-induced autonomic activation and changes in catecholamine levels are not mediated by changes in leptin levels in healthy humans. Clinical Endocrinology 2007; 66: 49–57

67 Rosenbaum M, et al. Effects of Weight Change on Plasma Leptin Concentrations and Energy Expenditure.

Journal of Clinical Endocrinology and Metabolism 197; 82: 3647–3654

Eat Stop Eat 193 68 Rosenbaum M et al. Low dose leptin administration reverses effects of sustained weight reduction on energy expenditure and circulating concentrations of thyroid hormones. The Journal of Clinical Endocrinology & Metabolism 87(5):2391–2394 69 Ahima RS, Flier JS. Leptin. Annual Review of Physiology. 2000; 62:413-37. 70 Kolaczynski JW, Considine RV, Ohannesian J, Marco C, Opentanova I, Nyce MR, Myint M, Caro JF. Responses of leptin to short-term fasting and refeeding in humans: a link with ketogenesis but not ketones themselves. Diabetes. 1996; 45(11):1511-5. 71 Brennan AM, Mantzoros CS. Drug insight: the role of leptin in human physiology and pathophysiology: emerging clinical applications in leptin deficient states. Nature Clinical Practice Endocrinology & Metabolism. 2006; 2:318–27. 72 Hislop MS, Ratanjee BD, Soule SG, Marais AD. Effects of anabolic–androgenic steroid use or gonadal testosterone suppression on serum leptin concentration in men. European Journal of Endocrinology 1999: 141; 40–46 73 Harle P, Straub RH. Leptin is a link between adipose tissue and inflammation. Annals of the New York

Academy of Sciences 2006; 1069: 454-462

74 Horio N et al. New frontiers in gut nutrient sensor research: nutrient sensors in the gastrointestinal tract: modulation of sweet taste sensitivity by leptin. J Pharmacol Sci. 112(1):8-12. 2010

75 Baker HWG, Santen RJ, Burger HG, De Krester DM, Hudson B, Pepperell RJ, Bardin CW. Rhythms in the secretion of gonadotropins and gonadal steroids. Journal of Steroids Biochemistry, 1975; 6:793-801.

76 Habito RC, Ball MJ (2001) Postprandial changes in sex hormones after meals of different composition. Metabolism 50:505–511 77 Habito RC, Montalto J, Leslie E, Ball MJ (2000) Effects of replacing meat with soyabean in the diet on sex hormone concentrations in healthy adult males. Br J Nutr 84:557– 563.

78 Meikle AW, Stringham JD, Woodward MG, Mcmurry MP (1990) Effects of a fat-containing meal on sex hormones in men. Metabolism 39:943–946. 79 Volek JS, Gomez AL, Love DM, Avery NG, Sharman MJ, Kraemer WJ (2001) Effects of a high-fat diet on postabsorptive and postprandial testosterone responses to a fat-rich meal. Metabolism 50:1351–1355.

80 Garrel DR, Todd KS, Pugeat MM, Calloway DH. Hormonal changes in normal men under marginally

negative energy balance. Am J Clin Nutr 1984;39:930-936.

81 Mohr BA, Bhasin S. Link CL, O'Donnell AB and McKinlay JB. The effect of changes in adiposity on testosterone levels in older men: longitudinal results from the Massachusetts Male Aging Study. European Journal of Endocrinology. 2006; 155:443-452.

82 Derby CA, Zilber S, Brambilla D, Morales KH, McKinlay JB. Body mass index, waist circumference and waist to hip ratio and change in sex steroid hormones: the Massachusetts Male Ageing Study. Clin Endocrinol (Oxf). 2006 Jul;65(1):125-31.

Eat Stop Eat 194 83 Strain GW, Zumoff B, Miller LK, Rosner W, Levit C, Kalin M, Hershcopf RJ, Rosenfeld RS. Effect of massive weight loss on hypothalamic-pituitary-gonadal function in obese men. J Clin Endocrinol Metab. 1988 May;66(5):1019-23. 84 Pritchard J, Després JP, Gagnon J, Tchernof A, Nadeau A, Tremblay A, Bouchard C. Plasma adrenal, gonadal, and conjugated steroids following long-term exercise-induced negative energy balance in identical twins. Metabolism. 1999 Sep;48(9):1120-7. 85 Khoo J, Piantadosi C, Worthley S, Wittert GA. Effects of a low-energy diet on sexual function and lower urinary tract symptoms in obese men. Int J Obes (Lond) 2010;34: 1396–403.

91

86 Cangemi R, Friedmann AJ, Holloszy JO, Fontana L, Long term effects of calorie restriction on serum sex-hormone concentrations in men. Aging Cell (2010) 9, 236-242

87 Friedl KE, Moore RJ, Hoyt RW, Marchitelli LJ, Martinez-Lopez LE, Askew EW. Endocrine markers of semistarvation in healthy lean men in a multistressor environment. J Appl Physiol. 2000 May;88(5):1820- 30

88 Röjdmark S. Influence of short-term fasting on the pituitary-testicular axis in normal men. Hormone Research. 1987; 25(3):140-6. 89 Bergendahl M, Aloi JA, Iranmanesh A, Mulligan TM, V eldhuis JD. Fasting suppresses pulsatile luteinizing hormone (LH) secretion and enhances orderliness of LH release in young but not older men. J Clin Endocrinol Metab. 1998 Jun;83(6):1967-75.

90 [Merck Manual 1992]. 91 Klibanski A, Beitins IZ, Badger T, Little R, McArthur JW. Reproductive function during fasting in men. Journal of Clinical Endocrinology and Metabolism. 1981; 53(2):258-63. 92 Chennaoui M, Desgorces F, Drogou C, Boudjemaa B, Tomaszewski A, Depiesse F, Burnat P, Chalabi H, Gomez-Merino D. Effects of Ramadan fasting on physical performance and metabolic, hormonal, and inflammatory parameters in middle-distance runners. Applied

Physiology Nutrition and Metabolism. 2009; 34(4):587-94. 93 Röjdmark S, Asplund A, Rössner S. Pituitary-testicular axis in obese men during short-term fasting. Acta Endocrinol (Copenh). 1989 Nov;121(5):727-32.

94 Klibanski A, Beitins IZ, Badger T, Little R, McArthur JW. Reproductive function during fasting in men. J Clin Endocrinol Metab. 1981 Aug;53(2):258-63. 95 Klibanski A, Beitins IZ, Badger T, Little R, McArthur JW. Reproductive function during fasting in men.*J Clin Endocrinol Metab* 53: 258, 1981

96 Roemmich JN and Sinning WE. Weight loss and wrestling training: effects on growth-related hormones. *J Appl Physiol* 82: 1760–1764, 1997. 97 Friedl KE, Moore RJ, Hoyt RW, Marchitelli LJ, Martinez-Lopez LE, Askew EW. Endocrine markers of semistarvation in healthy lean men in a multistressor environment. J Appl Physiol. 2000; 88(5): 1820–1830.

98 Hoehn K, Marieb EN (2010). *Human Anatomy & Physiology*. San Francisco: Benjamin Cummings. 99 Munck A, Naray-Fejes-Toth A. 1994. Glucocorticoids and stress: Permissive and suppressive actions. Ann

Eat Stop Eat 195 N Y Acad Sci 746: 115–130.

100 Bergendahl M, Vance ML, Iranmanesh A, Thorner MO, Veldhuis JD.Fasting as a metabolic stress

paradigm selectively amplifies cortisol secretory burst mass and delays the time of maximal nyctohemeral cortisol concentrations in healthy men. J Clin Endocrinol Metab. 1996 Feb;81(2):692-9.

101 Soeters MR. Intermittent fasting does not affect whole- body glucose, lipid, or protein metabolism. American Journal of Clinical Nutrition. 2009; 90:1244–51. 102 Schteingart DE, Gregerman RI, Conn JW. A comparison of the characteristics of increased adrenocortical function in obesity and Cushing's Syndrome. Metabolism 1963; 1:261-85.

103 Morton NM. Obesity and corticosteroids: 11beta-hydroxysteroid type 1 as a cause and therapeutic target in metabolic disease. *Mol Cell Endocrinol* 2010; 316: 154-164 104 Jacoangeli F, Zoli A, Taranto A, et al, 2002 Osteoporosis and anorexia nervosa: relative role of endocrine alterations and malnutrition. Eat Weight Disord 7: 190-195.

105 Guthrie HA. Introductory nutrition. 6th ed. St Louis Times Mirror/ Mosby College Publishing, 1986 106 Song WO, Chun OK, Obayashi S, Cho S, Chung CE. Is consumption of breakfast associated with body mass index in US adults? J Am Diet Assoc 2005 105(9): 1373-82 107 Gibson SA, O'Sullivan KR:

Breakfast cereal consumption patterns and nutrient intakes of British school children. J R Soc Health 115:336–370, 1995

108 Shlundt DG, Hill JO, Sbrocco T, Pope-Cordle J, Sharp T. The role of breakfast in the treatment of obesity: A randomized clinical trial. Am J Clin Nutr 1992;55:645-51 109 Cotton JR, Burley VJ, Blundell JE. Fat and satiety: No additional intensification of satiety following a fat supplement breakfast. Int J Obes, 1992 16(suppl 1): 11

110 Cotton JR, Burley VJ, Blundell JE: Fat and satiety - effect of fat in combination with either protein or carbohydrate. Obesity and Europe. Volume 93. London: J. Libbey; 1994:349-355.

111 Shlundt DG, Hill JO, Sbrocco T, Pope-Cordle J, Sharp T. The role of breakfast in the treatment of obesity: A randomized clinical trial. Am J Clin Nutr 1992;55:645-51 112 Morgan KJ, Zabik ME, Stampley GL. The role of breakfast in the diet adequacy of the U.S. adult population. J Am Coil Nutr 1986;5: 551-63.

113 Martin A, Normand S, Sothier M, Peyrat J, Louche- Pelissier C, Laville M. Is advice for breakfast consumption justified? Results from a short-term dietary and metabolic

experiment in young healthy men. British Journal of

Nutrition (2000) 84;337-344 114 Sarri KO, et al. Greek orthodox fasting rituals: a hidden characteristic of the Mediterranean diet of Crete. British Journal of Nutrition. 2004; 92: 277-284

115 Sarri KO, et al. Effects of Greek Orthodox Christian church fasting on serum lipids and obesity. BMC Public Health. 2003; 3: 3-16 116 Neel JV. Diabetes Mellitus: A "thrifty" genotype rendered detrimental by progress"? the American Journal of Human Genetics. 1962; 14:353-362.

Eat Stop Eat 196 117 Randle PJ, Garland PB, Hales CN, Newsholme EA, The glucose fatty-acid cycle. Its role in insulin sensitivity and the metabolic disturbances of diabetes mellitus. Lancet 1963:1;785-789. 118 Halberg N, et al. Effect of intermittent fasting and refeeding on insulin action in healthy men. Journal of Applied Physiology 2005; 99:2128-2136 119 Klein S, et al. Progressive Alterations in lipid and glucose metabolism during short-term fasting in young adult men. American Journal of Physiology 1993; 265 (Endocrinology and metabolism 28):E801-E806 120 Soules MR, Merriggiola MC, Steiner RA, Clifton DK, Toivola B, Bremner WJ. Short-Term fasting in normal women: absence of effects on gonadotrophin secretion and the menstrual cycle. Clinical Endocrinology 1994; 40:725- 731. 121 Hosker J, Matthews D, Rudenski A, Burnett M, Darling P, Bown E, Tu rner R: Continuous infusion of glucose with model assessment: measurement of insulin re s i s t a n c e and b-cell function in man. Diabetologia 28:401–411, 1985

122 Turner R, Holman R, Matthews D, Hockaday T, Peto J: Insulin deficiency and insulin resistance interaction in diabetes: estimation of their relative contribution by feedback analysis from basal plasma insulin and glucose concentrations. Metabolism 2 8 : 1086–1096, 1979

123 Matthews D, Hosker J, Rudenski A, Naylor B, Treacher D, Tu rner R: Homeostasis model assessment: insulin resistance and b-cell function from fasting plasma glucose and insulin concentrations in man. Diabetologia28:412–419, 1985

124 Wong MH, Holst C, Astrup A, Handjieva-Darlenska T, Jebb SA, Kafatos A, Kunesova M, Larsen TM, Martinez JA, Pfeiffer AF, van Baak MA, Saris WH, McNicholas PD, Mutch DM; DiOGenes. Caloric restriction induces changes in insulin and body weight measurements that are inversely associated with subsequent weight regain. PLoS One. 2012;7(8):e42858.

125 Svendsen PF, Jensen FK, Holst JJ, Haugaard SB,

Nilas L, Madsbad S. The effect of a very low calorie diet on insulin sensitivity, beta cell function, insulin clearance, incretin hormone secretion, androgen levels and body composition in obese young women.Scand J Clin Lab Invest. 2012 Sep;72(5):410-9.

126 Mason C, Foster-Schubert KE, Imayama I, Kong A, Xiao L, Bain C, Campbell KL, Wang CY, Duggan CR, Ulrich CM, Alfano CM, Blackburn GL, McTiernan A. Dietary weight loss and exercise effects on insulin resistance in postmenopausal women.Am J Prev Med. 2011 Oct;41(4):366-75. 127 Kassi E, Papavassiliou AG. Could glucose be a proaging factor? Journal of Cellular and Molecular medicine. 2008; 12(4):1194-8

128 Ling PR, Smith RJ, Bistrian BR. Acute effects of hyperglycemia and hyperinsulinemia on hepatic oxidative stress and the systemic inflammatory response in rats. Critical Care Medicine 2007; 35: 555-560.

129 Zechner R, Kienseberger PC, Hammerle G, Zimmermann R, Lass A. Adipose triglyceride lipase and the lipolytic catabolism of cellular fat stores. Journal of Lipid Research 2009;50:3-21.

130 Nielsen TS, Vandelbo MH, Jessen N, Pedersen SB, Jorgensen JO, Lund S, Moller N. Fasting, but not exercise, increases adipose triglyceride lipase (ATGL)

protein and

reduces G(0)/G(1) switch gene 2 (G0S2) protein and mRNA content in human adipose tissue. J Clin Endocrin Metab. 2011;96:E0000-E0000. Eat Stop Eat 197

131 Tunstall RJ, et al. Fasting activates the gene expression of UCP3 independent of genes necessary for lipid transport and oxidation in skeletal muscle. Biochemical and Biophysical Research Communications 2002; 294:301-308 132 Eakman GD, Dallas JS, Ponder SW, Keenan BS. The effects of testosterone and dihydrotestosterone on hypothalamic regulation of growth hormone secretion. *J Clin Endocrinol Metab* 81: 1217–1223, 1996.

133 Lang I, Schernthaner G, Pietschmann P, Kurz R, Stephenson JM, Templ H. Effects of sex and age on growth hormone response to growth hormone-releasing hormone in healthy individuals. *J Clin Endocrinol Metab* 65: 535–540, 1987.

134 Hartman ML, et al. Augmented growth hormone (GH) secretory burst frequency and amplitude mediate enhanced CH secretion during a two-day fast in normal men. Journal of Clinical Endocrinology and Metabolism 1992; 74(4):757-765

135 Vendelbo MH, Jorgensen JO, Pedersen SB,

Gormsen LC, Lund S, Schmitz O, Jessen N, and Moller N. Exercise and fasting activate growth hormone-dependent myocellular signal transducer and Activator of transcription-5b phosphorylation and Insulin-like growth factor-1 messenger ribonucleic acid expression in humans. Journal of Clinical Endocrinology and Metabolism. 2010; 95(9): 1-5

136 Rizza RA, Mandarino LJ & Gerich JE. Effects of growth hormone on insulin action in man. Mechanism of insulin resistance, impaired suppression of glucose production, and impaired stimulation of glucose utilization. Diabetes 1982 31 663–669

137 Norrelund H. Modulation of basal glucose metabolism and insulin sensitivity by growth hormone and free fatty acids during short-term fasting. European Journal of Endocrinology 2004; 150: 779-787

138 Hansen M, et al. Effects of 2 wk of GH administration on 24-h indirect calorimetry in young, healthy, lean men. American Journal of Physiology Endocrinology and Metabolism 2005; 289: E1030-E1038

139 Moller L, Dalman L, Norrelund H, Billestrup N, Frystyk J, Moller N, and Jorgensen JOL. Impact of fasting on growth hormone signaling and action in muscle and fat. Journal of Clinical Endocrinology and Metabolism. 2009;4:

965-972.

140 Szego CM, White A. The influence of purified growth hormone on fasting metabolism. J Clin Endocrinol Metab 8;1948:594. 141 Norrelund H. The protein-retaining effects of growth hormone during fasting involve inhibition of muscle- protein breakdown. Diabetes 2001;50:96-104

142 Norrelund H, Rils AL, Moller N. Effects of GH on protein metabolism during dietary restriction in man. Growth hormone & IGF Research 2002; 12: 198-207 143 Moller N, Jorgensen JO. Effects of growth hormone on glucose, lipid and protein metabolism in human subjects. Endocrine Reviews. 2009; 30:152-177

144 Norrelund H. Abstracts of Ph.D. Dissertations – Effects of growth hormone on protein metabolism during dietary restriction. Studies in Normal, GH-Deficient and Obese Subjects. Danish Medical Bulletin 2001; 47 (5): 370 145 Norrelund H. The metabolic role of growth hormone in humans with particular reference to fasting. Growth Hormone and IGF research. 2005;15:95-122.

Eat Stop Eat 198 146 Oscarsson J, Ottosson M, Eden S. Effects of growth hormone on lipoprotein lipase and hepatic lipase. J Endocrinol Invest 22; 1999: 2-9 147 Oscarsson J, Ottosson M, Vikman-adolfsson K, et al. GH but not IFG-1 or insulin increases lipprotein lipase activity in muscle tissues of hpophysectomizes rats. J Endocrinol. 160;1999:247-255. 148 Veldhuis JD, Iranmanesh A, Ho KK, Waters MJ, Johnson ML, Lizarralde G. Dual defects in pulsatile growth hormone secretion and clearance subserve the hyposomatotropism of obesity in man. J Clin Endocrinol Metab. 1991 Jan;72(1):51-9.

149 Cornford AS, Barkan AL, Horowitz JF. Rapid suppression of Growth Hormone concentration by overeating: Potential mediation by hyperinsulinemia. J Clin Endocrinol Metab 96: 824-830, 2011.

150 Rabinowitz D, Zierler KL. A metabolic regulating device based on the actions of growth hormone and of insulin singly and together in the human forearm 1963. Nature; 199: 913-915.

151 Veldhuis JD, Roemmich JN, Richmond EJ, Bowers CY. Somatotropic and gonadotropic axes linkages in infancy, childhood, and the pubertyadult transition. *Endocr Rev* 27: 101–140, 2006.

152 Veldhuis JD. Aging and hormones of the hypothalamo- pituitary axis: gonadotropic axis in men and somatotropic axes in men and women. Ageing Research Reviews. 2008; 7: 189–208.

153 Finkelstein JW, Roffwarg HP, Boyar RM,

Kream J, Hellman L. Age-related change in the twenty-
four- hour

spontaneous secretion of growth hormone. Journal of
Clinical Endocrinolology and Metabolism. 1972
Nov;35(5):665-70 154 Corpas E, Harman SM, Blackman
MR. Human growth hormone and human aging. Endocrine
Reviews. 1993; 14: 20–39.

155 Frayne, K.N. 1993. Insulin resistance and lipid
metabolism. *Curr. Opin. Lipidol.* **4**:197–204 156 Boden,
G., Chen, X., Ruiz, J., White, J.V., and Rosetti, L. 1994.
Mechanism of fatty acid induced

inhibition of glucose uptake. *J. Clin. Invest.* **93**:2438–
2446. 157 Kanaley JA, Weatherup-Dentes MM, Jaynes EB,
Hartman ML. Obesity attenuates the growth hormone
response to exercise. Journal of Clinical Endocrinology
Metabolism. 1999;84:3156-3161.

158 Redman LM, Veldhuis JD, Rood J, Smith SR,
Williamson D, Ravussin E; Pennington CALERIE Team.
The effect of caloric restriction interventions on growth
hormone secretion in nonobese men and women. Aging
Cell. 2010 Feb;9(1):32-9.

159 Rasmussen MH, Hvidberg A, Juul A, et al.
Massive weight loss restores 24-hour growth hormone
release profiles and serum insulin-like growth factor-I

levels in obese subjects. Journal of Clinical Endocrinology Metabolism. 1999; 80:1407-1415

160 Mauras N, O'brien KO, Welch S, et al. Insulin-like growth factor 1 and growth hormone (GH) treatment in GH-Deficient humans: differential effects on protein, glucose, lipid and calcium metabolism. J Clin Endocrinol Metab 85;2000:1686-1694.

161 Rennie MJ. Claims for the anabolic effects of growth hormone: a case of the Emperor's new clothes? British Journal of Sports Medicine 2003; 37:100–105 Eat Stop Eat 199

162 Duncan GG, Cristofori FC, Yue JK, Murthy MSJ: Control of obesity by intermittent fasts. Med Clin N Amer 48: 1359, 1964. 163Johnstone, AM. Fasting – the ultimate diet? Obesity Reviews 2007; 8(3): 211-222

164 Lionetti L, Mollica MP, Lombardi A, Cavaliere G, Gifuni G, Barletta A. From chronic overnutrition to insulin resistance: the role of fat-storing capacity and inflammation. Nutriton, Metabolism & Cardiovascular disease 2009;19:146-152.

165 Chung HY, Kim HJ, Kim JW, Yu BP. The inflammation hypothesis of aging: molecular modulation by calorie restriction. Annals of the New York Academy of Sciences. 2001; 928:327-35.

166 Senn JJ, Klover PJ, Nowak IA, and Moony RA. IL-6 Induces Cellular Insulin Resistance in Hepatocytes. Diabetes. 2002; 51(12):3391-9. 167 Bharat B. Aggarwal, R.V. Vijayalekshmi, and Bokyung Sung. Targeting Inflammatory Pathways for Prevention and Therapy of Cancer: Short-Term Friend, Long-Term Foe. Clinical Cancer Research 2009; 15(2): 425-430.

168 Kershaw EE, Flier JS. Adipose tissue as an endocrine organ. Journal of Clinical Endocrinology and Metabolism. 2004; 89:2548–2556. 169 Loffreda S, Yang SQ, Lin HZ, Karp CL, Brengman ML, Wang DJ, Klein AS, Bulkley GB, Bao C, Noble PW, Lane MD, Diehl AM. Leptin regulates proinflammatory immune responses. Federation of American Societies for Experimental Biology Journal. 1998 Jan;12(1):57-65.

170 Esposito K, Nappo F, Marfella R, Giugliano G, Giugliano F, Ciotola M, Quagliaro L, Ceriello A, Giugliano D. Inflammatory cytokine concentrations are acutely increased by hyperglycemia in humans: role of oxidative stress. Circulation. 2002 Oct 15;106(16):2067-72.

171 Dixit VD. Adipose-immune interactions during obesity and caloric restriction: reciprocal mechanisms regulating immunity and health span. Journal of Leukocyte Biology. 2008: 84:882-892.

172 Morgan TE, Wong AM, and Finch CE. Anti-inflammatory mechanisms of dietary restriction in slowing aging processes. Interdisciplinary Topics in Gerontology. 2007; 35:83-97.

173 Fontana L. Neuroendocrine factors in the regulations of inflammation: Excessive adiposity and caloir restriction. Experimental Gerontology. 2009; 44:41-45. 174 Prestes J, Shiguemoto G, Botero JP, Frollini A, Dias R, Leite R, et al. Effects of resistance training on resistin, leptin, cytokines, and muscle force in elderly post-menopausal women. Journal of Sports Science. 2009 27(14):1607-1615.

175 Bruun JM, Helge JW, Richelsen B, Stallknecht B. Diet and exercise reduce low-grade inflammation and macrophage infiltration in adipose tissue but not in skeletal muscle in severely obese subjects. American Journal of Physiology Endocrinology and Metabolism. 2006 May;290(5):E961-7.

176 Schapp LA, Plijm SMF, Deeg DJh and Visser M. Inflammatory markers and loss of muscle mass (Sarcopenia) and strength. 2006. American Journal of Medicine; 199: U82-U90.

Eat Stop Eat 200 177 Toth MH, Mattews DE, Tracy RP and Previs MJ. Age- related differences in skeletal muscle protein synthesis:

relation to markers of immune activation. American Journal of Pysiology Endocrinology and Metabolism 2005; 288:E883-E891. 178 Visser M, Pahor M, Taaffe DR, Goodpaster BH, Simonsick EM, Newman AB et al. Relationship of interluekin-6 and tumor necrosis factor-α with muscle mass and muscle strength in elderly men ad women" The health ABC study. Journal of Gerontology Series A: Biological Science and Medical Science 2002; 57: M326-M332.

179 Deter RL, De Duve C. Influence of glucagon, an inducer of cellular autophagy, on some physical properties of rat liver lysosomes. J Cell Biol 1967;33:437–449 180 A.M. Cuervo, E. Bergamini, U.T. Brunk, W. Droge, M. Ffrench, A. Terman, Autophagy and aging: the importance of maintaining ''clean'' cells, Autophagy 1 (2005) 131e140.

181 T Kanazawa, Ikue Taneike, Ryuichiro Akaishi, Fumiaki Yoshizawa, Norihiko Furuya, Shinobu Fujimura, and Motoni Kadowaki. Amino Acids and Insulin Control Autophagic Proteolysis through Different Signaling Pathways in Relation to mTOR in Isolated Rat Hepatocytes. THE JOURNAL OF BIOLOGICAL CHEMISTRY Vol. 279, No. 9, Issue of February 27, pp.

8452–8459, 2004

182 Glynn EL, Fry CS, Drummond MJ, Timmerman KL, Dhanani S, Volpi E, Rasmussen BB. Excess leucine intake enhances muscle anabolic signaling but not net protein anabolism in young men and women. J Nutr. 2010 Nov;140(11):1970-6.

183 Joon-Ho Sheen, Roberto Zoncu, Dohoon Kim, David M. Sabatini Defective Regulation of Autophagy upon Leucine Deprivation Reveals a Targetable Liability of Human Melanoma Cells In Vitro and In Vivo. Cancer Cell, Volume 19, Issue 5, 613-628, 17 May 2011

184 Ding, WX. The emerging role of autophagy in alcoholic liver disease Exp Biol Med 1 May 2011: 546-556.

185 Hara T, et al. Suppression of basal autophagy in neural cells causes neurodegenerative disease in mice. Nature 2006; 441:885-9

186 Komatsu M, et al. Loss of autophagy in the central nervous system causes neurodegeneration in mice. Nature 2006; 441:880-4   187 Mizushima N, Levine B, Cuervo AM, Klionsky DJ. Autophagy fights disease through cellular self- digestion. Nature 2008; 451:1069-75

188 Alirezaei M, Kiosses WB, Flynn CT, Brady NR, Fox HS. Disruption of neuronal autophagy by infected microglia results in neurodegeneration. PLoS ONE 2008;

3:2906

189 Orvedahl A, Levine B. Eating the enemy within: autophagy in infectious diseases. Cell Death Differ 2009; 16:57-69 190 Alirezaei M, Kemball CC, Flynn CT, Wood MR, Whitton JL, Kiosses WB. Short-term fasting induces profound neuronal autophagy. Autophagy. 2010 Aug;6(6):702-10.

191 Hara, N., K. Nakamura, M. Matsui, A. Yamamato, Y. Nakahara, R. Suzuki-Migishima, M. Y okoyama, K. Mishima, I. Saito, H. Okana, and N. Mizushima. Suppression of basal autophagy in neural cells causes neurodegenerative disease in mice. Nature. In press

192 Komatsu M, et al. Loss of autophagy in the central nervous system causes neurodegeneration in mice. Nature 2006; 441:880-4 Eat Stop Eat 201

193 Jaeger PA, Wyss-Coray T. All-you-can-eat: autophagy in neurodegeneration and neuroprotection. Mol Neurodegener 2009; 4:16 194 Hung SY, Huang WP, Liou HC, Fu WM. Autophagy protects neuron from Aβ-induced cytotoxicity. Autophagy 2009; 5:502-10.

195 Donati A, Cavallini G., Paradiso C., Vittorini S., Pollera M., Gori Z. and E. B. Age-related changes in the autophagic proteolysis of rat isolated liver cells: effects of antiaging dietary restrictions. J Gerontol A Biol Sci

Med Sci. 2001; 56: B375-383. 196 Rubinsztein DC. The roles of intracellular protein- degradation pathways in neurodegeneration. Nature. 2006; 443: 780-786

197 K. Kirkegaard, M.P. Taylor, W.T. Jackson, Cellular autophagy: surrender, avoidance and subversion by microorganisms, Nat. Rev. Microbiol. 2 (2004) 301e314

198 B. Levine, Eating oneself and uninvited guests: autophagy-related pathways in cellular defense, Cell 120 (2005) 159e162

199 M. Ogawa, C. Sasakawa, Bacterial evasion of the autophagic defense system, Curr. Opin. Microbiol. 9 (2006) 62e68 200 M.S. Swanson, Autophagy: eating for good health, J. Immunol. 177 (2006) 4945e4951.

201 Anson RM, et al. Intermittent fasting dissociates beneficial effects of dietary restriction on glucose metabolism and neuronal resistance to injury from calorie intake. Proc Natl Acad Sci USA 2003; 100:6216- 20

202 Duan W, et al. Dietary restriction normalizes glucose metabolism and BDNF levels, slows disease progression, and increases survival in huntingting mutant mice. Proc Natl Acad Sci USA 2003; 100:2911-6

203 Tohyama D, Yamaguchi A and Yamashita T. Inhibition of a eukaryotic initiation factor (eIF2Bdelta/F11A3.2) during adulthood extends lifespan in

Caenorhabditis elegans. FASEB J. 2008; 22: 4327-4337

204 Nair U, Klionsky DJ. Activation of autophagy is required for muscle homeostasis during physical exercise. Autophagy. 2011 Dec 1;7(12).

205 Sandri M. Autophagy in health and disease. 3. Involvement of autophagy in muscle atrophy. Am J Physiol Cell Physiol 2010; 298:C1291-7 206 Drummond DA. Mistranslation-induced protein misfolding as a dominant constraint on coding-sequence evolution. Cell. 2008; 134: 341-352

207 Fishebin L, Biological effects of Dietary Restriction. Springer-Verlag, New York.1991. 208 Lane MA, Ingram DK, Roth GS. Caloric Restriction in nonhuman primates: Effects on Diabetes and cardiovascular disease risk. Toxilogical Sciences 1999; 52s: 41-48.

209 Varaday KA, Bhutani S, Church EC, Klempel EC, Short-term modified alternate-day fasting: a novel dietary strategy for weight loss and cardioprotection in obese adults. American Journal of Clinical Nutrition 2009; 90:1138–43.

Eat Stop Eat 202

210 Stirling LJ, Yeomans MR. Effect of exposure to a forbidden food on eating in restrained and unrestrained

women. Int J Eat Disord 35: 59–68, 2004 211 Rogers PJ, Smit HJ. Food craving and food "addiction": A critical review of the evidence from a biopsycholsocial perspective. Pharmacology Biochemistry and Behavior, Vol. 66, No. 1, pp. 3–14, 2000

212 Bernard, C. *Lecon de Physiologie Expdrirnentale Appliqute* ci *la Midecine. faites au College de France. Tome IeTC: ours du semester d'hiver 1854-1855.* J.-B. BailliBre, Paris, 1855.

213 Randle PJ, Garland PB, Hales CN, and Newsholme EA. The glucose fatty-acid cycle. Its role in insulin sensitivity and the metabolic disturbances of diabetes mellitus. *Lancet* 1: 785-789, 1963.

214 Vendelbo MH, Clasen BF, Treebak JT, Møller L, Krusenstjerna- Hafstrøm T, Madsen M, Nielsen TS, Stødkilde-Jørgensen H, Pedersen SB, Jørgensen JO, Goodyear LJ, Wojtaszewski JF, Møller N, Jessen N. Insulin resistance after a 72-h fast is associated with impaired AS160 phosphorylation and accumulation of lipid and glycogen in human skeletal muscle. Am J Physiol Endocrinol Metab 302: E190– E200, 2012.

215 Nilsson LH, and Hultman E. Liver glycogen in man-- the effect of total starvation or a carbohydrate-poor diet

followed by carbohydrate refeeding. *Scand J Clin Lab Invest* 32: 325-330, 1973. 216 Green JG, Johnson NA, Sachinwalla T, Cunningham CW, Thompson MW, Stannard SR. Moderate- intensity endurance exercise prevents short-term starvation-induced intramyocellular lipid accumulation but not insulin resistance. *Metabolism* 60: 1051–1057, 2011.

217 Johnson NA, Stannard SR, Rowlands DS, Chapman PG, Thompson CH, O'Connor H, Sachinwalla T, Thompson MW. Effect of shortterm starvation versus high-fat diet on intramyocellular triglyceride accumulation and insulin resistance in physically fit men. *Exp Physiol* 91: 693–703, 2006.

218 Bergman BC, Cornier MA, Horton TJ, Bessesen DH. Effects of fasting on insulin action and glucose kinetics in lean and obese men and women. *Am J Physiol Endocrinol Metab* 293: E1103–E1111, 2007.

219 Bergman BC, Cornier MA, Horton TJ, Bessesen DH. Effects of fasting on insulin action and glucose kinetics in lean and obese men and women. *Am J Physiol Endocrinol Metab* 293: E1103–E1111, 2007.

220 Dominici FP, Argentino DP, Bartke A, Turyn D (2003) The dwarf mutation decreases high dose insulin responses in skeletal muscle, the opposite of effects in

liver. Mech Ageing Dev 124:819 – 827

221 Salih DA, Brunet A (2008) FoxO transcription factors in the maintenance of cellular homeostasis during aging. Curr Opin Cell Biol 20:126 –136 222 Food in Early Modern Europe, Ken Albala [Greenwood Press:Westport CT] 2003 (p. 232)

223 Rituals of Dinner, Margaret Visser [Penguin Books:New York] 1991 (p. 158-9) 224 Herman CP, Mack D. Restrained and unrestrained eating. Journal of personality. 1975;43:647-660.

225 Herman CP, Polivy J. The self-regulation of eating. Journal of Personality 1992; 43: 647-660. 226 Knight LJ, Boland FJ. Restrained eating: An experimental disentragnelment of the disinhibition variables of perceived calories and food type. Journal of Abnormal psychology 1989:98;412-420.

227 Westenhoefer J, Stunkard AJ, Pudel V. Validation of the flexible and rigid control dimesions of dietary restraing. International journal of Eating Disorders 1999;26: 53-64. Eat Stop Eat 203

228 Halberg N, Henriksen M, Soderhamn N, et al. Effect of intermittent fasting and refeeding on insulin action healthy men. Journal of Applied Physiology 2005; 99:2128-2136 229 Carlson HE, Shah JH. Aspartame and its

constituent amino acids: effects on prolactin, cortisol, growth hormone,

insulin, and glucose in normal humans. American Journal of Clinical Nutrition. 1989: 49; 427-32 230 Okuno G, Kawakami F, Tako H, Kashihara T, Shibamoto S, Yamazaki T, Yamamoto K, Saeki M. Glucose tolerance, blood lipid, insulin and glucagon concentration after single or continuous administration of aspartame in diabetics. Diabetes Research and Clinical Practice1986 Apr; 2(1):23-7.

231 Petrie HJ, Chown SE, Belfie LM, Duncan AM, McLaren DH, Conquer JA, Graham TE. Caffeine ingestion increases the insulin response to an oral-glucose-tolerance test in obese men before and after weight loss. American Journal of Clinical Nutrition. 2004 Jul;80(1):22-8.

232 Graham TE, Sathasivam P, Rowland M, Marko N, Greer F, Battram D. Caffeine ingestion elevates plasma insulin response in humans during an oral glucose tolerance test. Canadian Journal of Physiology and Pharmacology 2001 Jul;79(7):559-65.

233 Ho KY , Evans WS, Blizzard RM, V eldhuis JD, Merriam GR, Samojlik E, Furlanetto R, Rogol AD, Kaiser DL, Thorner MO. 1987. Effects of sex and age on the 24-hour profile of growth hormone secretion in man:

importance of endogenous estradiol concentrations. J Clin Endocrinol Metab 64:51–58.

234 Yen SSC, Vela P, Rankin J, Littell AS. 1970 Hormonal relationships during the menstrual cycle. JAMA. 211:1513– 1517. 235 Devesa J, Lois N, Arce V, Diaz MJ, Lima L, Tresguerres JA. 1991 The role of sexual steroids in the modulation of growth hormone (GH) secretion in humans. J Steroid Biochem Mol Biol. 40:165–173.

236 Veldhuis J.D. et al. Relative effects of estrogen, age, and visceral fat on pulsatile growth hormone secretion in healthy women. Am J Phsiol Endocrinol Metab 297: E367- E74, 2009.

237 Weltman A, Weltman JY, Hartman ML, et al. 1994 Relationship between age, percentage body fat, fitness and 24-hour growth hormone release in healthy young adults: effects of gender. J Clin Endocrinol Metab. 78:543–548. 238 Wennink JMB, Delemarre-van de Waal HA, Schoemaker R, Blaauw G, van den Brakern C, Schoemaker J. 1991 Growth hormone secretion patterns in relation to LH and estradiol secretion throughout normal female puberty. ActaEndocrinol (Copenh). 124:129 –135.

239 Frantz AG, Rabkin MT. 1965 Effects of estrogen and sex difference on secretion of human growth hormone. J Clin Endocrinol Metab. 25:1470 –1480.

240 Merimee TJ, Fineberg SE. 1971 Studies of the sex- based variation of human growth hormone secretion. J Clin Endocrinol Metab. 33:896 –902. 241 Heilbronn LK, Civitarese AE, Bogacka I, Smith ST, Hulver M, Ravussin E. Glucose tolerance and skeletal muscle gene expression in response to alternate day fasting. Obse Res. 2005; 13:574-581.

242 Warren MP, Vande Wiele RL. 1973 Clinical and metabolic features of anorexia nervosa. Am J Obstet Gynecol. 117:435– 449. Eat Stop Eat 204

243 Frisch RE, Wyshak G, Vincent L. 1980 Delayed menarche and amenorrhea in ballet dancers. N Engl J Med. 303:17–19. 244 Frisch, RE, McArthur. 1974 Menstrual cycles: fatness as a determinant of minimum weight for height necessary for their maintenance or onset. Science. 185:949

245 Friedl KE, et al. Lower limit of body fat in healthy active men. J ApplPhsiol 77(2): 933-940, 1994 246 Thong, Farah S. L., Cyndy McLean, and Terry E. Graham. Plasma leptin in female athletes: relationship with body fat, reproductive, nutritional, and endocrine factors. *J Appl Physiol* 88: 2037–2044, 2000.

247 Azizi F. Effect of Dietary Composition on Fasting- Induced Changes in Serum Thyroid Hormones and

Thyrotropin Metabolism, Vol. 27, NO. 8 (August), 1978

248 Borissova AM, Tankova T, Kirilov G, Koev D 2005 Gender-dependent effect of ageing on peripheral insulin action. Int J Clin Pract 59:422–426

249 Paula FJ, Pimenta WP, Saad MJ, Paccola GM, Piccinato CE, Foss MC 1990 Sex-related differences in peripheral glucose metabolism in normal subjects. Diabetes Metab 16:234–239

250 Soeters MR, Sauerwein HP, Groener JE, Aerts JM, Ackermans MT, Glatz JF, Fliers E, Serlie MJ.Gender-related differences in the metabolic response to fasting.J Clin Endocrinol Metab. 2007 Sep;92(9):3646-52. Epub 2007 Jun 12.

251 Bergman BC, Cornier M-A, Horton TJ, Bessesen DH. Effects of fasting on insulin action and glucose kinetics in lean and obese men and women. *Am J Physiol Endocrinol Metab* 293: E1103–E1111, 2007.

252 Lado-Abeal J, Prieto D, Lorenzo M, Lojo S, Febrero M, Camarero E, Cabezas-Cerrato J. Differences between men and women as regards the effects of protein-energy malnutrition on the hypothalamic- pituitary-gonadal axis. Nutrition. 1999 May;15(5):351-8.

253 Mittendorfer B, Horowitz JF, Klein S. Gender differences in lipid and glucose kinetics during short-term

fasting. *Am J Physiol Endocrinol Metab* 281: E1333–E1339, 2001.

254 Soeters MR, Sauerwein HP, Groener JE, Aerts JM, Ackermans MT, Glatz JF, Fliers E, Serlie MJ. Gender-related differences in the metabolic response to fasting. *J Clin Endocrinol Metab* 92: 3646–3652, 2007.

255 Kiens , B. , C. Roepstorff , J. F. Glatz , A. Bonen , P. Schjerling , J. Knudsen , and J. N. Nielsen . 2004 . Lipid- binding proteins and lipoprotein lipase activity in human skeletal muscle: infl uence of physical activity and gender. *J. Appl. Physiol.* 97 : 1209 – 1218 .

256 Klempel MC, Kroeger CM, Bhutani S, Trepanowski JF, Varady KA.Intermittent fasting combined with calorie restriction is effective for weight loss and cardio-protection in obese women.Nutr J. 2012 Nov 21;11:98.

257 Harvie MN, Pegington M, Mattson MP, Frystyk J, Dillon B, Evans G, Cuzick J, Jebb SA, Martin B, Cutler RG, Son TG, Maudsley S, Carlson OD, Egan JM, Flyvbjerg A, Howell A.The effects of intermittent or continuous energy restriction on weight loss and metabolic disease risk markers: a randomized trial in young overweight women. Int J Obes (Lond). 2011 May;35(5):714-27.

258 Data tabulated from VenusIndex.com Eat Stop Eat 205 259 Exercise AC. Ace Lifestyle & Weight Management Consultant Manual, The Ultimate Resource for Fitness Professionals. American Council on Exercise; 2009. 260 Alvero R, Kimzey L, Sebring N, Reynolds J, Loughran M, Nieman L, Olson BR.Effects of fasting on neuroendocrine function and follicle development in lean women.J Clin Endocrinol Metab. 1998 Jan;83(1):76-80. 261 Olson BR, Cartledge T, Sebring N, Defensor R, Nieman L. 1995 Short-term fasting affects luteinizing hormone secretory dynamics but not reproductive function in normal-weight sedentary women. J Clin Endocrinol Metab. 80:1187–1193. 262 *Klibanski A, Beitins IZ, Badger T, Little R, McArthur JW.Reproductive function during fasting in men. J Clin Endocrinol Metab. 1981 Aug;53(2):258-63.* 263 Friedl KE et al. Endocrine markers of semistarvation in healthy lean men in a multistressor environment. J Appl Physiol 88:1820-1830, 2000. 264 Dye L, Blundell JE. Menstrual cycle and appetite control: implications for weight regulation. Hum Reprod 1997;12:1142-51.

265 Van Vugt DA. Brain imaging studies of appetite in the context of obesity and the menstrual cycle. Hum

Reprod Update 2010;16:276–92. 266 Asarian L, Geary N. Modulation of appetite by gonadal steroid hormones. Philos Trans R Soc Lond B Biol Sci 2006;361:1251–63.

267 Alonso-Alonso M, Ziemke F, Magkos F, Barrios FA, e al.Brain responses to food images during the early and late follicular phase of the menstrual cycle in healthy young women: relation to fasting and feeding.Am J Clin Nutr. 2011 Aug;94(2):377-84.

268 Goldberg AL, Etlinger JD, Goldspink DF, Jablecki C. Mechanism of work-induced hypertrophy of skeletal muscle. Medicine and Science in Sports Exercise. 1975 7:248-61.

269 Bean J, Frontera W. Strength and Power Training. Harvard Health Publications. 2008 270 Hausenblas HA, Falloon EA. Exercise and body image: A meta analysis. Psychology and health. 2006; 21: 33-47.

271 Wernbom M, Augustsson J and Thome´e R. The Influence of Frequency, Intensity, Volume and Mode of Strength Training on Whole Muscle Cross-Sectional Area in Humans. Sports Medicine 2007; 37 (3): 225- 264

272 Burd NA, West DWD, Staples AW, et al. Low-Load high volume resistance exercise stimulates muscle protein synthesis more than high-load low volume resistance exercise in young men. Plos One. 2010; 5(8):

e12033

273 Dishman RK. 1988 Exercise adherence: its impact on public health. Champaign Il: Human Kinetics. 274 Niven A, Rendell E, Chisholm L. Effects of 72-h of exercise abstinence on affect and body dissatisfaction in healthy female regular exercisers. Journal of Sports Sciences, 2008; 26(11): 1235-1242

Eat Stop Eat 206 275 Benjamin R. The Surgeon General's Vision for a Healthy and Fit Nation. Rockville, MD: U.S. Department of Health and Human Ser- vices, Public Health Service, Office of the Surgeon General; 2010. 276 Kiens B. Effect of endurance training on fatty acid metabolism: local adaptations. *Med Sci Sports Exercise* 29: 640–645, 1997. 277 Kiens B. Effect of endurance training on fatty acid metabolism: local adaptations. *Med Sci Sports Exercise* 29: 640–645, 1997. 278 Kiens B and Lithell H. Lipoprotein metabolism influenced by training-induced changes in human skeletal muscle. *J Clin Invest* 83: 558–564, 1989.

279 Blundell JE, Stubbs RJ, Hughes DA, Whybrow S, King NA. Cross-talk between physical activity and appetite control: does PA stimulate appetite? Proc Nutr Soc 2003; 62: 651–661.

280 Whybrow S, Hughes DA, Ritz P, Johnstone AM,

Horgan GW, King N et al. The effect of an incremental increase in exercise on appetite, eating behavior and energy balance in lean men and women feeding ad libitum. Br J Nutr 2008; 100: 1109–1115.

281 Unick JL, Otto AD, Goodpaster BH, Helsel DL, Pellegrini CA, Jakicic JM. The acute effect of walking on energy intake in overweight/obese women. Appetite 2010; 55: 413–419.

282 Pendleton VR, Goodrick GK, Poston WS, Reeves RS, Foreyt JP. Exercise augments the effects of cognitive- behavioral therapy in the treatment of binge eating. Int J Eat Disord 2002;31:172–84.

283 Martins C, Morgan L, Truby H. A review of the effects of exercise on appetite regulation: an obesity perspective. Int J Obes 2008; 32: 1337–1347. 284 Thompson D, Karpe F, Lafontan M, Frayn K. Physical activity and exercise in the regulation of human adipose tissue physiology. Physiol Rev. 2012 Jan;92(1):157-91

285 Ismail I, Keating SE, Baker MK, Johnson NA. A systematic review and meta-analysis of the effect of aerobic vs. resistance exercise training on visceral fat. Obes Rev. 2012 Jan;13(1):68-91. 286 Slentz CA, Bateman LA, Willis LH, Shields AT, Tanner CJ,et al. Effects of aerobic vs. resistance training on visceral and liver fat stores, liver

123

enzymes, and insulin resistance by HOMA in overweight adults from STRRIDE AT/RT. Am J Physiol Endocrinol Metab. 2011 Nov;301(5):E1033-9.

287 Jacoangeli F, Zoli A, Taranto A, et al, 2002 Osteoporosis and anorexia nervosa: relative role of endocrine alterations and malnutrition. Eat Weight Disord 7: 190-195.

288 Henson J, Yates T, Biddle SJ, Edwardson CL, Khunti K, Wilmot EG, Gray LJ, Gorely T, Nimmo MA, Davies MJ. Associations of objectively measured sedentary behaviour and physical activity with markers of cardiometabolic health.Diabetologia. 2013 May;56(5):1012-20.

289 Prestes J, Shiguemoto G, Botero JP, Frollini A, Dias R, Leite R, et al. Effects of resistance training on resistin, leptin, cytokines, and muscle force in elderly post-menopausal women. Journal of Sports Science 2009 27(14):1607-1615

290 Bruunsgaard H. Physical activity and modulation of systemic low-level inflammation J Leukoc Biol 78: 819-835, 2005. Eat Stop Eat 207

291 Timmerman KL, Flynn MG, Coen PM, Markofski MM and Pence BD. Exercise training-induced lowering of inflammatory (CD14+CD16+) monocytes: a

role in the anti-inflammatory influence of exercise? Journal of Leukocyte Biology. 2008;84:1271-1278.)

292 Bean J, Frontera W. Strength and Power Training. Harvard Health Publications. 2008 293 Hausenblas HA, Falloon EA. Exercise and body image: A meta analysis. Psychology and health. 2006. 21; 33-47.

294 Ulen GC, Huizinga MM, Beecb B, Elasy TA. Weight regain prevention. Clinical Diabetes. 2008;26:100-113. 295 Delbridge EA, Prendergast LA, Pritchard JE, Proietto J. One-Year weight maintenance after significant weight loss in healthy overweight and obese subjects: does diet composition matter? American Journal of Clinical Nutrition 2009; 90:12093-13.

296 Foster GD, Wyatt HR, Hill JO, et al. A randomized trial of a low-carbohydrate diet for obesity. New England Journal of Medicine 2003;348:2082-90.

297 Dansinger ML, Gleason JA, Griffith JL, et al. Comparison of the Atkins, Ornish, Weight Watchers, and Zone diets for weight loss and heart diseases risk reduction: A randomized trial. Journal of the American Medical Association 2005; 293:43-53.

298 Russell J de Souza, George A Bray, Vincent J Carey, et al. Effects of 4 weight-loss diets differing in fat, protein, and carbohydrate on fat mass, lean mass, visceral

adipose tissue, and hepatic fat: results from the POUNDS LOST trial. Am J Clin Nutr 2012;95:614–25.

299 Vogels N, Westerterp-Plantenga MS. Successful Long- term weight Maintenance: A 2-year follow up. Obesity: 15(5);2007 1258-1266 300 Westenhoefer J, Stunkard AJ, Pudel V. Validation of the flexible and rigid control dimensions of dietary restraint. Int J Eat Disord 1999;26:53–64.

301 Provencher V, Drapeau V, Tremblay A, Despres JP, Lemieux S. Eating behaviors and indexes of body composition in men and women from the Quebec family study. Obes Res 2003;11:783–92.

302 Drapeau V, Provencher V, Lemieux S, Despres JP, Bouchard C, Tremblay A. Do changes in eating behaviors predict changes in body weight? Results from the Quebec Family Study. Int J Obes Relat Metab Disord 2003;27:808– 14.

303 McGuire MT, Jeffery RW, French SA, Hannan PJ. The relationship between restraint and weight and weight- related behaviors among individuals in a community weight gain prevention trial. Int J Obes Relat Metab Disord 2001;25:574–80.

304 Provencher V, Begin C, Tremblay A, Mongeau L, Boivin S, Lemieux S. Short-term effects of a ''health-at-

every-size'' approach on eating behaviors and appetite ratings. Obesity 2007;15:957 66.

305 Teixeira PJ, Silva MN, Coutinho SR, Palmeira AL, Mata J, Vieira PN, et al. Mediators of weight loss and weight loss maintenance in middle-aged women. Obesity 2009, 281.

306Johnstone, AM. Fasting – the ultimate diet? Obesity Reviews 2007; 8(3): 211-222 Eat Stop Eat 208 307 Clarke, Paul A. B.; Andrew Linzey (1996). Dictionary of ethics, theology and society. Routledge Reference. Taylor & Francis. p. 58

308 Fatouros I, Chatzinikolaou A, Paltoglou G, et al. Acute resistance exercise results in catecholaminergic rather than hypothalamic–pituitary–adrenal axis stimulation during exercise in young men Stress: The International Journal on the Biology of Stress (October 2010), 13 (6), pg. 461-468

309 Mastorakos G et al.Exercise as stress model and the interplay between the hypothalamus-pituitary- adrenal and the hypothalamus-pituitary-thyroid axes Horm Metab Res , v.37 , p.577 , 2005

310 Kazushige Goto, Kohei Shioda, and Sunao Uchida. Effect of 2 days of intensive resistance training on appetite- related hormone and anabolic hormone responses

Clin Physiol Funct Imaging (2013) 33, pp131– 136

311 Kuipers H. Training and overtraining: an introduction. Med Sci Sports Exerc (1998); 30: 1137– 1139. 312 Jacoangeli F, Zoli A, Taranto A, et al, 2002 Osteoporosis and anorexia nervosa: relative role of endocrine alterations and malnutrition. Eat Weight Disord 7: 190-195.

313 Phillips SM, Tipton KD, Aarsland A, Wolf SE, Wolfe RR. Mixed muscle protein synthesis and breakdown after resistance exercise in humans. Am J Physiol Endocrinol Metab 273: E99–E107, 1997.

314 Dreyer HC, Fujita S, Cadenas JG, Chinkes DL, Volpi E, Rasmussen BB. Resistance exercise increases AMPK activity and reduces 4E-BP1 phosphorylation and protein synthesis in human skeletal muscle. J Physiol 576: 613– 624, 2006.

315 Fujita S, Dreyer HC, Drummond MJ, Glynn EL, Volpi E, Rasmussen BB. Essential amino acid and carbohydrate

ingestion prior to resistance exercise does not enhance post- exercise muscle protein synthesis. J Appl Physiol. In press. 316 Rennie MJ, Edwards RH, Halliday D, Matthews DE, Wolman SL, Millward DJ. Muscle protein synthesis measured by stable isotope techniques in man: the effects of feeding and fasting. *Clin Sci (Lond)* 63: 519– 523, 1982. 317 Biolo G, Tipton KD, Klein S, Wolfe RR. An abundant supply of amino acids enhances the metabolic effect of exercise on muscle protein. *Am J Physiol Endocrinol Metab* 273: E122–E129, 1997.

318 Kiens B, Roepstorff C, Glatz JF, Bonen A, Schjerling P, Knudsen J, and Nielsen JN. Lipid-binding proteins and lipoprotein lipase activity in human skeletal muscle: influence of physical activity and gender. *J Appl Physiol* 97: 1209–1218, 2004.

319 Epel ES. Psychological and metabolic stress: A recipe for accelerated cellular aging? Hormones 2009; 8(1):7-22 320 Rutters F, Nieuwenhuizen AG, Lemmens SG, Born JM, Westerterp-Plantenga MS, 2009 Hyperactivity of the HPA axis is related to dietary restraint in normal weight women. Physiol Behav 96: 315-319.

321 Vigersky RA, Anderson AE, Thompson RH, and Loriaux DL. Hypothalamic dysfunction in secondary amenorrhea associated with simple weight loss. *N Engl J Med* 297: 1141–1145, 1977.

322 Ursin H, Baade E, and Levine S. (Editors). *Psychobiology of Stress. A Study of Coping Men.* New York: Academic, 1978. Eat Stop Eat 209

323 Mosek A, Korczyn AD. Fasting headache,

weight loss, and dehydration. Headache 1999; 29: 225-227 324 Dresher MJ, Elstein Y. Prophylactic COX 2 inhibitor: An end to the yom kippur headache. Headache 2006; 26: 1487-1491

325 Soules MR, Merriggiola MC, Steiner RA, Clifton DK, Tiovala B, Bremmer WJ. Short-term fasting in normal women: absence of effects on gonadotrophin secretion and he menstrual cycle. Clin Endocrinol 1994;40(6):725-31

326 Olson BR, Cartledge T, Sebring N, Defensor R, Neiman L. Short-term fasting affects luteinizing hormone secretory dynamics but not reproductive function in normal-weight sedentary women. J Clin Endocrinol Metab. 1995;80(4):1187-93.

327 Alverno R, Kimzey L, Sebring N, Reynolds J, Loughran M, Nieman L, Olson BR. Effects of fasting of neurendocrine function and follicle development in lean women. J Clin Endocrinology and Metabolism, 1998; 83(1):76-80.

328Mattson MP, Duan w, Guo Z. Meal size and frequency affect neuronal plasticity and vulnerability to disease: cellular and molecular mechanisms. Journal of Neurochemistry 2003; 84(3): 417-431 329 Bhasin S, Cryer PE, Vigersky R. The hormone Foundations Patient guide

130

on the diagnosis and management of hypoglycemic disorders (low Blood Sugar) in adults. The hormone Foundation, 2009.

330 Alkén J, Petriczko E, Marcus C. Effect of fasting on young adults who have symptoms of hypoglycemia in the absence of frequent meals. European Journal of Clinical Nutrition. 2008 Jun;62(6):721-6.

331 Johnson JB, Summer W, Cutler RG et al. Alternate day calorie restriction improves clinical findings and reduces markers of oxidative stress and inflammation in overweight adults with moderate asthma. Free Radical Biology & Medicine 2007; 42: 665-674

332 Aksungar FB, Topkaya AE, Akyildiz M. Interlukin-6, C-reactive protein and biochemical parameters during prolonged intermittent fasting. Annals of Nutrition and Metabolism 2007; 51:88-95

333 Martin B, Mattson MP, Maudsley S. Caloric Restriction and intermittent fasting: Two potential diets for successful brain aging. Ageing Research Reviews 2006; 5: 332-353.

334 Funada J, Dennis AL, Roberts R, Karpe F, Frayn KN. Regulation of subcutaneous adipose tissue blood flow is related to measures of vascular and autonomic function. Clinical Science. 2010; 119(8):313-322. 335 Trappe TA,

White F, Lambert CP, Cesar D, Hellerstein M, Evans WJ. Effect of ibuprofen and acetaminophen on postexercise muscle protein synthesis. American Journal of Physiology Endocrinology Metabolism. 2002 Mar;282(3):E551-6.

336 Krentz JR, Quest B, Farthing JP, Quest DW, Chilibeck PD. The effects of ibuprofen on muscle hypertrophy, strength, and soreness during resistance training. Applied Physiology Nutrition Metabolism. 2008 Jun;33(3):470-5. 337 Hall MN. mTOR-what does it do? Transplant Proc. 2008; 40: S5-8

338 Duffey KJ and Popkin BM. Energy Density, Portion Size, and Eating Occasions: Contributions to Increased Energy Intake in the United States 2011 Jun;8(6):e1001050.

Eat Stop Eat 210 339 Safdie FM, Dorff T, Quinn D, Fontana L, Wei M, et al. Fasting and cancer treatment in humans: A case report. Aging. 2009;1(12):1-20
Brad Pilon is the author of Eat Stop Eat, and one of the top experts on the science of fasting, including the widely misunderstood protocol of intermittent fasting. Brad has a Master's Degree in Applied Human Nutrition, and years of experience in the supplement industry as a Research Analyst and Development Manager. His personal blog, Eat Blog Eat, is a valuable resource for the research on fasting and information for how to optimize and troubleshoot

132

fasting diet protocols, and his workout programs and books are designed to educate people on the truth about how to utilize fasting to achieve the results they want.

Made in the USA
Lexington, KY
25 August 2017